Women and Depression

The purpose of this book is to present a spectrum of women's experiences with depression. The book is unique in presenting both qualitative and quantitative studies on various stages of women's experiences with depression including its psychological and social antecedents, its adverse consequences, and the impact of psychological and community interventions. Our aim has been to present some of the recurrent themes and vital links in this chain of experiences. One such common theme has to do with the importance of acquiring and maintaining control over the evaluation of self-worth by the individual. Stressful circumstances and the negative social encounters may produce the greatest harm and consequent depression by depriving individuals' control over the processes involved in the evaluation of self-worth.

This book will be of interest to clinical psychologists, counsellors, psychiatrists, mental health practitioners and community service providers.

This book was published as a special issue of the *Journal of Prevention and Intervention in the Community.*

Peter Horvath is Professor and Clinical Program Co-ordinator in the Department of Psychology, Acadia University in Wolfville, Nova Scotia, Canada. Dr Horvath is a Registered Psychologist in Nova Scotia and engages in part-time clinical practice. His research has been published in various journals including *Psychological Bulletin*, the *Journal of Consulting and Clinical Psychology*, and *Canadian Psychology* among others.

Women and Depression

Antecedents, Consequences, and Interventions

Edited by Peter Horvath

Routledge
Taylor & Francis Group
LONDON AND NEW YORK

First published 2009 by Routledge

2 Park Square, Milton Park, Abingdon, Oxfordshire OX14 4RN
605 Third Avenue, New York, NY 10017

Routledge is an imprint of the Taylor & Francis Group, an informa business

First issued in hardback 2020

Typeset in Times by Value Chain, India

British Library Cataloguing in Publication Data
A catalogue record for this book is available from the British Library

ISBN13: 978-0-7890-3662-9 (hbk)
ISBN13: 978-0-7890-3663-6 (pbk)

CONTENTS

Introduction: Women, Depression, and the Struggle for Control Over the Evaluation of Self-Worth

Peter Horvath, PhD

Stressful life circumstances, among other psychosocial factors, are important contributors to depression in women (Mazure, Keita, & Blehar, 2002). However, they may not be the primary antecedents of depression. A key finding of past research is that depression-prone individuals experience difficulties in the control and regulation of their self-worth (Roberts & Monroe, 1999). Depressed women tend to adopt socially-derived and externally-imposed cognitive constructs or frames of reference (i.e., goals and evaluation criteria) by which they evaluate their self-worth (Jack & Dill, 1992). Research findings support this view (Moretti, Rein, & Wiebe, 1998). Social expectations and social power determine which cognitive constructs or frames of reference we use to evaluate ourselves (Jack, 1999). Consistent with this proposition, the studies in this issue suggest that women who are vulnerable for depression are trapped within a particular frame of reference whereby the self is seen as rejected, subordinate, and a passive victim of hostile circumstances rather than as a free and wilful agent. Depressed women lose the social struggle for control of the frames of reference by which they evaluate the self. Such notions go beyond psychological constructs such as learned helplessness in contextualizing the origins of vulnerability for depression. Vulnerable individuals are unable to resist the devaluation of their self-worth by the use of externally imposed social categories.

The findings of the studies in this issue have implications for effective psychological, social, and community interventions for depression in general, and depressed women in particular. In addition to attempting to remove the stressors and negative views that precipitate depression, psychological interventions need to encourage and empower individuals to own and control the processes of self-evaluation. One way to do this is to support individuals to choose and own the frames of reference by which they determine their self-worth. Education in the schools and public education in the community should not only encourage achievement and personal success but also should teach individuals that they are in charge when it comes to evaluating their worth as persons. Community agencies and groups need to consider whether their interventions support individuals to acquire control over frames of reference by which they evaluate themselves or whether intentionally or unintentionally they evoke social processes that are alien or harmful to the person's sense of worth. Community interventions need to assist individuals in ways whereby they not only retain their dignity as human beings but are also encouraged to have control over the assistance they receive. The movement toward community-centered interventions for mental health problems is likely to facilitate such an empowering process (Horvath, Bissix, MacLeod, & Barr, 2005). This approach involves collaborative and cooperative efforts by community services and agencies to make more grass-roots resources and services available and to place interventions as much as possible under the control of the individuals who need the assistance. Under such conditions, not only women but also all individuals with emotional problems are more likely to evaluate themselves as persons of worth.

In sum, stressful circumstances and negative social encounters may produce the greatest harm and consequent depression when they deprive the individual control over the processes of self-evaluation. In contrast, the best psychological and community interventions may be those that help to restore and maintain this control.

REFERENCES

Horvath, P., Bissix, G., MacLeod, K., & Barr, C. (2005). Community services and resources for depressed women in two rural regions of Nova Scotia. [On-line serial] *Journal of Rural and Community Development, 1*, 18-31.

Jack, D. C. (1999). Silencing the self: Inner dialogues and outer realities. In T. Joiner & J. C. Coyne (Eds.), *The interactional nature of depression: Advances in interpersonal approaches* (pp. 221-246). Washington, DC: American Psychological Association.

Jack, D. C., & Dill, D. (1992). The Silencing the Self Scale: Schemas of intimacy associated with depression in women. *Psychology of Women Quarterly, 16*, 97-106.

Mazure, C. M., Keita, G. P., & Blehar, M. C. (2002). *Summit on women and depression: Proceedings and recommendations.* Washington, DC: American Psychological Association. (Available online at: http://www.apa.org/pi/wpo/women&depression.pdf).

Moretti, M. M., Rein, A. S., & Wiebe, V. J. (1998). Relational self-regulation: Gender differences in risk for dysphoria. *Canadian Journal of Behavioural Science, 30*, 243-252.

Roberts, J. E., & Monroe, S. M. (1999). Vulnerable self-esteem and social processes in depression: Toward an interpersonal model of self-esteem regulation. In T. Joiner & J. C. Coyne (Eds.), *The interactional nature of depression: Advances in interpersonal approaches* (pp. 149-187). Washington, DC: American Psychological Association.

Self-Silencing, Anger and Depressive Symptoms in Women: Implications for Prevention and Intervention

Josephine Tan, PhD

Brooke Carfagnini, MA

INTRODUCTION

The predominance of women among the depressed (Bebbington, 1996; Benazzi, 2000) has generated several explanations to account for the sex differential. One of the more recent explanations is the silencing the self theory (STS; Jack, 1991) which postulates that more women than men are depressed because of their greater tendency to self-silence in intimate relationships in order to preserve harmony and the relationship and to adhere to the traditional female role. Self-silencing, which involves the concealment of one's true feelings from others, can lead to a sense of divided self wherein the compliant self that is presented on the outside is incongruent with the personal feelings on the inside. The sense of divided self might be accompanied by feelings of anger and self-condemnation that can lead to heightened vulnerability for depression in some women (Jack, 1999). Self-silencing is undertaken to decrease interpersonal conflict in the relationship out of fear of retaliation and to adhere to idealized images of women as loving and responsible for the emotional climate of the relationship (Jack, 1991; Jack & Dill, 1992).

Gender-specific prohibitions against displays of anger and aggression in females further discourage the expression of such feelings (Jack, 1999). Women are socialized to place a strong emphasis on relationships as they are a central component of the female sex role identity and emotional activity. Failure to attain and maintain intimate ties can result in feelings of shame, guilt, and depression (Gilligan, 1993; Jack, 1991; Kaplan, 1986).

Jack (1991) noted that despite the depressed woman's tendency towards active self-silencing and anger suppression, rage and frustration would sometimes erupt, often inappropriately expressed or displaced towards innocent others such as children. The consequences of such anger expression, including negating responses from a spouse and increased self-condemnation, would tend to further erase hopes for relationship improvement and provide additional impetus for continued self-silencing behaviours, in turn predicting depression vulnerability.

Although research on Jack's model is relatively limited, the results show some support. Greater self-silencing in women has been found to relate to greater depression (Cramer, Gallant, & Langlois, 2005; Jack & Dill, 1992; Page, Stevens, & Galvin, 1996; Thompson, Whiffen, & Aube, 2001), less marital satisfaction (Thompson, 1995), and greater perception of marital partner as critical or intolerant (Thompson et al., 2001). A mixed-sex study reported that greater self-silencing was correlated with greater fear of anger expression and with greater anger suppression and that previously-depressed individuals self-silenced more than the never-depressed (Brody, Hagga, Kirk, & Solomon, 1999). Self-concealment which reflects a tendency to hide distressing personal information from others (Kelly & Achter, 1995) was shown to mediate the link between self-silencing and depression (Cramer et al., 2005). Finally, feminine sex role type was found to be positively correlated with anger suppression, which in turn was reported to be the best predictor of high depressive symptoms (Kopper & Epperson, 1996).

Furthering our understanding of the psychological factors that are associated with depression in women has implications for addressing a wide-spread health problem in the community. Depression is the most common mental disorder (Desjarlais, Eisenberg, Good, & Kleinman, 1995) and strikes 1 out of every 5 women (Kessler et al., 1994). It occurs more frequently in women than in men, regardless whether it is indexed by elevated depressive symptoms or diagnosed clinical disorder (Nolen-Hoeksema, 1995). Le, MuZoz, Ippen, and Stoddard (2003) noted the importance for mental health initiatives to go beyond treatment and argued for a national priority to be placed on the prevention of depression in women. Others have called for prevention efforts to focus on subclinical depression or elevated depressive symptoms (Clarke, DeBar, Lynch, & Wisdom, 2003; Gillam, 2003; Parks & Herman, 2003) because it presents a risk factor for major depression (Clarke et al., 1995, 2001). As well, the psychosocial impairment associated with elevated depressive symptoms has been reported to be nearly comparable to that associated with clinical depression (Gotlib, Lewinsohn, & Seeley, 1995).

Following the same argument that subclinical depression warrants attention, the present study examined Jack's silencing the self theory with a group of women who presented with varying severity of depressive symptoms in order to determine the role of self-silencing in intimate relationships, anger expression and anger suppression in predicting the severity of depressive symptoms. In addition, the presence of strong social and cultural components in self-silencing would lend itself to community prevention and intervention approaches. It was expected that higher depression severity would be predicted by greater self-silencing, anger expression and anger suppression. Additional analyses were also performed on two sub-samples, high depression and low depression groups that were derived from the full sample to assess for differences in self-silencing, anger expression and anger suppression between women with no depression and those with elevated depressive symptoms.

METHOD

Participants

Out of the 60 questionnaires that were mailed to women who responded to recruitment efforts, 57 were completed and returned, yielding a 95% response rate. Responses from one woman were excluded from the data analysis because she suffered from a neurological medical condition that might contribute to her depressive symptoms. The final sample for the study consisted of 56 women (age *M* = 36.34 years, *SD* = 11.09) who were currently living with an intimate partner, and were free of chronic physical or neuropsychological problems that could contribute to their depression symptoms. Seventeen women were in treatment for depression. With the exception of three Asian women, all participants were Caucasians which approximates the ethnic ratio of Asian: Caucasian residents in the community from which the sample was drawn. The depression severity, as measured with the Beck Depression Inventory-II (BDI-II, Beck, Steer, & Brown, 1996), ranged from 0 to 39 (*M* = 12.93, *SD* = 10.19) in the sample.

Measures

Beck Depression Inventory-II (BDI-II; Beck et al., 1996). The BDI-II is a widely used measure of current depression severity. Its 21 items reflect the DSM-IV-TR (American Psychiatric Association, 2000) criteria of behavioural, cognitive, and somatic-vegetative symptoms that are responded to on a severity scale ranging from 0 to 3. The range of possible scores is 0 to 63 with higher numbers indicating greater severity of depressive symptoms. The interpretive guidelines for the BDI-II for patients with major depression are 0-13 (minimal depression), 14-19 (mild depression), 20-28 (moderate depression), and 29-63 (severe depression). Lower cut-off threshold is recommended to detect depression and minimize the number of false negatives (Beck et al., 1996). The BDI-II has been shown to have excellent psychometric properties in research with psychiatric and nonpsychiatric populations (Beck, Steer, & Garbin, 1988). The internal consistency of the BDI-II in the present study was .92.

Silencing the Self Scale (STSS; Jack, 1991). This 31-item scale uses a 5-point response scale (1 = strongly disagree, 5 = strongly agree) to measure beliefs and behaviours about self-expression within one's intimate relationship. It yields a global self-silencing score that ranges from 31 to 155 with higher scores indicating greater self-silencing. The STSS has good internal consistency ranging from .86 to .94 (Jack & Dill, 1992; Smolak & Munstertieger, 2002; Thompson, 1995) and good construct validity and test-retest reliability (Jack & Dill, 1992). It has four subscales that are based on the themes of self-silencing derived from Jack's (1991) work with depressed women. The Externalized Self-Perception subscale which contains six items reflects the degree to which one judges the self by external standards. The Care as Self-Sacrifice subscale has nine items and assesses the degree to which one puts the needs of others before the self. The Silencing the Self subscale is composed of nine items and looks at the degree to which one inhibits self-expression and action to avoid conflict, possible loss, and retaliation from others. Finally, the Divided Self subscale has seven items and examines the degree to which one presents an outer compliant self that does not express internal authentic thoughts and feelings. In the present study, the Cronbach's alpha was .92 for the STSS full scale, .77 for the Externalized Self-Perception subscale, .73 for the Care as Self-Sacrifice subscale, .89 for the Silencing the Self subscale, and .86 for the Divided Self subscale.

State-Trait Anger Expression Inventory-2 (STAXI-2; Spielberger, 1999). The STAXI-2 was designed to provide a measurement of the experience, control, and expression of anger. It yields a total of six scales of which two are relevant to the present study. The Anger Expression-Out scale (AX-O) has eight items with possible scores ranging from 8 to 32 and assesses the frequency that angry feelings are expressed in verbally or physically aggressive behaviour. The Anger Expression-In scale (AX-I) similarly is composed of eight items with possible scores ranging from 8 to 32 and measures how often angry feelings are felt but not expressed. Items on both the AX-O and AX-I scales are responded to on a 4-point scale that ranges from 1 (almost never) to 4 (almost always). In the present study, the Cronbach's alpha was computed to be .83 for AX-O and .75 for AX-I.

Procedure

Recruitment for this study was conducted as part of the recruitment efforts for a larger project that looked at the meanings that men and women ascribe to the act of self-silencing. Participants were recruited from several health care sources and the general community through advertisements in the media (newspapers, television), and posters posted in public areas and health care facilities. The present study was promoted as a research project that examines psychological functioning and perception of selves within intimate relationships. Those who responded to the recruitments efforts were given information about the study and its procedure. A copy of the research questionnaire was then mailed out to each of them with instructions to complete and return it within one week of receipt. The study was conducted in strict adherence to the Tri-Council Research Ethics guidelines.

Design and Analysis

The main analyses conducted on the full sample consisted of correlational analysis to determine associations among the measures, and stepwise regression techniques to determine which of the measures predicted the BDI-II scores. Additional analyses were undertaken to compare high and low depression groups. The full sample was split approximately three-way based on the severity of the BDI-II scores. The bottom third (low depression group) consisted of 20 women with BDI scores no greater than 7 ($M = 3.00$, $SD = 2.29$, range = 0 to 7). The top third (high depression group) was composed of 20 women with BDI scores of 16 or higher ($M = 24.20$, $SD = 7.23$, range = 16 to 39). The remaining 17 women were excluded from the analyses. Fourteen women (70%) in the high depression group were currently in treatment as opposed to two (10%) in the low depression group. All participants were Caucasians in both groups with the exception of three Asian women in the high depression group. There was no significant difference in age between the high depression ($M = 38.00$ years, $SD = 9.89$) and low depression ($M = 35.55$ years, $SD = 12.47$) group.

RESULTS

Correlational Analysis

Table 1 presents the correlations among the measures and their subscales. The results indicated that both BDI-II and AX-I were positively and significantly associated with AX-O, STSS full scale and its four subscales Externalized Self-Perception, Care as Self-Sacrifice, Silencing the Self, and Divided Self. BDI-II scores also showed a significant positive correlation with AX-I. Not surprisingly, the four STSS subscales were significantly intercorrelated and correlated with the STSS full scale score.

Stepwise Regression

Stepwise regression was conducted on the BDI-II with AX-I and AX-O as predictor variables. The results showed that only AX-I contributed significantly to the prediction of the BDI-II, $\Delta R^2 = .47$, $\Delta F(1, 54) = 47.28$, $p < .001$.

A separate stepwise regression was conducted on the BDI-II with the four STSS subscales as predictor variables. Results showed that both the Externalized Self-Perception subscale, $\Delta R^2 = .38$, $\Delta F(1, 54) = 33.47$, $p < .001$, and to a lesser extent the Silencing the Self subscale, $\Delta R^2 = .05$, $\Delta F(1, 53) = 4.49$, $p < .05$, contributed to the prediction of the BDI-II.

TABLE 1. Pooled Correlations Among BDI-II, STSS and Its Subscales, and the Anger Scales

Measure	1	2	3	4	5	6	7	8
1. BDI-II	—	.56**	.62**	.29*	.41**	.46**	.34**	.68**
2. STSS full scale		—	.74**	.70**	.79**	.85**	–.01	.51**
3. Externalized Self-Perception			—	.49**	.33*	.58**	.22	.55**
4. Care as Self-Sacrifice				—	.33*	.39**	.02	.29*
5. Silencing the Self					—	.64**	–.24	.30*
6. Divided Self						—	.05	.48**
7. AX-O							—	.43**
8. AX-I								—

Note. BDI-II = Beck Depression Inventory - II, STSS = Silencing the Self Scale, AX-O = Anger Expression-Out, AX-I = Anger Expression-In.

*$p < .05$. **$p < .01$.

Multivariate Analyses

To determine whether there were significant differences between the high and low depression group on the anger scales, a MANOVA was carried out. There was a significant multivariate effect, $F(2, 37) = 13.21, p < .001, \eta^2 = .42$, power > .99. Follow-up univariate F-tests were conducted separately on the two anger scales to determine which scale contributed to the significant multivariate effect. To keep the overall Type I error rate at .05, the Bonferroni adjustment was used in which the .05 alpha rate was divided between the two tests. Hence, each of the F-tests was assessed at a more stringent p-value of 0.025 (= .05/2). The results showed that AX-I [$F(1,38) = 27.05, p < .001, \eta^2 = .42$, power > .99] contributed to group differences. The test for AX-O revealed a near significance, $F(1, 38) = 5.27$, $p = .027$, $\eta^2 = .12$, power = .61. An examination of the group means showed that the high depression group scored higher on both anger scales than did the low depression group (see Table 2).

Similarly, a MANOVA was carried out with the four STSS subscales. A significant omnibus multivariate effect was found, $F(4, 35) = 10.96$, $p < .001$, $\eta^2 = .56$, power > .99. As before, separate univariate F-tests were performed on each of the STSS subscales using the Bonferroni adjustment in which the overall alpha level of .05 was divided among the four tests, resulting in each test being assessed against the more stringent

Table 2. Pooled and Within-Group Means (Standard Deviations) for High and Low Depression Groups on BDI-II, STSS and Its Subscales, and the Anger Scales

Variables	High Depression (n = 20)	Low Depression (n = 20)	Pooled Sample (n = 56)
BDI-II	24.20 (7.23)	3.00 (2.29)	12.93 (10.19)
STSS full scale	99.30 (18.04)	65.60 (17.18)	82.14 (21.93)
Externalized Self-Perception	23.00 (4.29)	14.30 (4.33)	18.21 (5.69)
Care as Self-Sacrifice	27.35 (7.48)	20.80 (6.01)	24.23 (6.86)
Silencing the Self	27.05 (8.51)	18.00 (5.97)	22.21 (8.57)
Divided Self	21.90 (6.27)	12.50 (5.45)	17.48 (7.26)
AX- O	19.20 (5.73)	15.85 (3.13)	17.98 (5.27)
AX-I	21.40 (4.85)	14.60 (3.27)	18.04 (5.06)

Note. BDI-II = Beck Depression Inventory-II, STSS = Silencing the Self Scale, AX-O = Anger Expression-Out, AX-I = Anger Expression-In.

p level of .0125. Results revealed that all four subscales, Externalized Self-Perception [$F(1, 38) = 40.73, p < .001, \eta^2 = .52$, power > .99], Care as Self-Sacrifice [$F(1, 38) = 9.32, p < .01, \eta^2 = .20$, power = .85], Silencing the Self [$F(1, 38) = 15.16, p < .001, \eta^2 = .29$, power = .97], and Divided Self [$F(1, 38) = 25.58, p < .001, \eta^2 = .40$, power > .99] contributed to group separation. The high depression group scored higher than the low depression group on all four subscales (see Table 2).

DISCUSSION

The pattern of findings supports Jack's silencing the self theory. As expected, women who reported greater depression severity also tended to report greater anger expression, anger suppression and self-silencing in general. The observation that anger expression and anger suppression can occur in the same individual may seem paradoxical. However, it makes sense if one accepts that anger suppression will eventually lead to anger expression if the anger is not channeled through other more adaptive means such as effective and assertive communication.

When the predictive utility of the measures and their subscales were investigated, it was found that only anger suppression and the two STSS subscales, Externalized Self-Perception and Silencing the Self, predicted depression severity. Hence women who are at risk for depression in intimate relationships are more likely to suppress their anger, judge themselves by external standards, and inhibit their words and actions to avoid conflict with others.

When the women were divided into two groups reflecting high and low depression severity, it was found that the high depression group tended to suppress their anger to a greater degree. They also relied on external standards to judge themselves, sacrificed their needs for others, hid their true selves from others, and experienced a disparity between their inner and outer selves. In other words, they ascribed more to the traditional female sex role.

The present findings provide some possible suggestions for interventions with depressed women with particular emphasis on the predictor variables found in the study. Depression has been postulated to reflect masked anger in women (e.g., Gordon & Allen, 1990). Ascription to such a position has led some to advocate the expression of anger as an intervention strategy for with women in counselling (Gilbert, 1980; Wills-Brandon, 1989). Assisting depressed women to become more assertive and effective in expressing negative thoughts and emotions might serve to minimize self-silencing, narrow the disparity between the inner and outer selves, and decrease anger suppression and sense of hopelessness in the relationship. This in turn might favour effective problem resolution and subsequent alleviation of depressive symptoms. However, asserting one's self is not necessarily prescriptive for all relationships–it might endanger the woman in abusive situations where there is a power imbalance in the relationship and where the abusive partner might view the woman's self-assertion as a challenge to his/her authority.

Cognitive work might also be conducted to assist the women to rely more on their internal values in evaluating themselves than on externally imposed standards on how they should feel or behave. This might involve identifying and challenging traditional sex role beliefs about a woman's role and behaviour in intimate relationships that contribute to the depression, coupled with an understanding of the societal factors that contribute to the maintenance of those beliefs and behaviour. Interventions that incorporate the consideration of such factors are made possible with mental health service providers who are cognizant of the part that sex-role socialization might play in depression in women and who are vigilant in assessing women for self-silencing. In such cases where self-silencing is a factor in the depression, the women would need to question aspects of the traditional female sex role that bind them to self-sacrifice and learn to adopt a more balanced perspective where their own selves also matter.

Preventive interventions could be undertaken on a larger societal level through psychoeducational strategies in schools and in the community that focus on improving assertive and effective communication and anger management. Given that sex-role socialization begins at a very young age, schools present a pivotal place for intervention.

Community-based mental health promotion projects that are developed in collaboration with local communities, educational institutions, health agencies and authorities, and workplaces in order to reach a wider range of the population could serve to increase public awareness of depression and its link to self-silencing and anger management, and to increase public access to interventions that focus on treatment of depression, communication skills and assertiveness training. The public also needs to be cognizant of any biases that they might hold against women who disclose, especially their anger and frustration.

Jack (1991) wrote that historically, women have self-silenced because of social and economic inequality. Given that women generally tend to be at an economic disadvantage in society (Harvey, 1999; Rollins, 1996), community efforts to assist these women to become more financially independent of others might give them the freedom to speak up for themselves.

Although working on an individual, group or community level can be beneficial to help women with depression, the key to this whole issue is a societal change in the socialization of women and attitudes towards women. Both men and women need to learn that caring for one's self in addition to others is not selfish, that expressing one's inner thoughts effectively might help in problem resolution, and that one's inner values need to be considered in self-evaluation instead of blind obedience to societal expectations of how a woman should behave.

The findings of the present study have to be considered within its methodological drawbacks. The study had a small sample size derived from community and clinical populations which limits the generalizability of its results to either population. The cut-off score on the BDI-II to define the high depression group was derived on the basis of dividing the full sample into thirds, and not directed by the interpretive guidelines of the BDI-II. The low depression group consisted of women who were all not depressed, as defined by the BDI-II interpretive guidelines. The high depression group, however, consisted of women whose BDI-II scores ranged from mild to severe of whom 14 were diagnosed with major depression and the remaining 6 were not. The heterogeneity of the research participants as defined by the range of their depressive scores and the sampling from both community and clinical populations could have implications for the testing of Jack's theory that was originally developed with women with clinical depression. It would have been informative to compare a true clinical sample (elevated depression scores + major depression diagnosis) with a subclinical sample (elevated depression scores only) to determine whether Jack's model apply to both. Additionally, it is possible that the sampling was not random in that there might have been important differences, such as in the degree of self-silencing or self-concealment, between the women in the study and those who did not volunteer for participation. As well, the self-report measures used in the study are subjective by nature and not necessarily accurate. Other facets of data collection procedures such as corroborating reports from third parties might increase the validity of the findings. Finally, the sample was drawn from a relatively rural community that limits its application to urban populations.

In conclusion, the results from the present study support Jack's silencing the self theory and identified anger suppression along with two facets of self-silencing (judging the self according to external standards and hiding one's true self from others) to be predictors of elevated depressive symptoms in women. It needs to be acknowledged that depression has several associated features, including biological factors, and that self-silencing and anger suppression are two of many aspects that need to be considered. Future research can address an interesting question that arises from the present study: Would adopting a more balanced perspective of women's roles in relationships be a protective factor against depression, and what aspects of such sex role beliefs are involved? As well, the efficacy of assertive communication skills in addressing female depression with different populations (e.g., students, workers, patients) has to be assessed. Finally, examining women who are non-depressed might provide a clue as to their protective factors. Encouraging more research efforts in this area would provide evidence that is required to secure government funding for intervention and prevention projects in the community.

REFERENCES

American Psychiatric Association. (2000). *Diagnostic and statistical manual of mental disorder* (4th ed., text rev.). Washington, DC: Author.

Bebbington, P. (1996). The origins of sex differences in depressive disorder: Bridging the gap. *International Review of Psychiatry*, *8*, 295-332.

Beck, A. T., Steer, R. A., & Brown, G. R. (1996). *Beck Depression Inventory: Manual.* San Antonio, Texas: The Psychological Corporation.

Beck, A. T., Steer, R. A., & Garbin, M. G. (1988). Psychometric properties of the Beck Depression Inventory: Twenty-five years of evaluation. *Clinical Psychology Review*, *8*, 77-100.

Benazzi, F. (2000). Female vs. male outpatient depression: A 448-case study in private practice. *Progress in Neuro-Psychopharmacology and Biological Psychiatry*, *24*, 475-481.

Brody, C. L., Hagga, D. A. F., Kirk, L., & Solomon, A. (1999). Experiences of anger in people who have recovered from depression and never-depressed people. *Journal of Nervous and Mental Disease*, *187*, 400-405.

Clarke, G., DeBar, L., Lynch, F., & Wisdom, J. (2003). Issues in the prevention of depression in women: A commentary on Le, MuZoz, Ippen, and Stoddard (2003). *Prevention and Treatment*, *6*, 202-210.

Clarke, G. N., Hawkins, W., Murphy, M., Sheeber, L. B., Lewinsohn, P. M., & Seeley, J. R. (1995). Targeted prevention of unipolar depressive disorder in an at-risk sample of high school adolescents: A randomized trial of a group cognitive intervention. *Journal of the American Academy of Child and Adolescent Psychiatry*, *34*, 312-321.

Clarke, G. N., Hornbrook, M., Lynch, F., Polen, M., Gale, J., & Beardslee, W. (2001). A randomized trial of a group cognitive intervention for preventing depression in adolescent offspring of depressed parents. *Archives of General Psychiatry*, *58*, 1127-1134.

Cramer, K. M., Gallant, M. D., & Langlois, M. W. (2005). Self-silencing and depression in women and men: Comparative structural equation models. *Personality and Individual Differences, 39*, 581-592.

Desjarlais, R., Eisenberg, L., Good, B., & Kleinman, A. (1995). *World mental health: Problems and priorities in low-income countries.* New York, NY: Oxford University Press.

Gilbert, L. A. (1980). Feminist therapy. In A. M. Brodsky & R. T. Hare-Mustin (Eds.), *Women and psychotherapy* (pp. 245-265). New York, NY: Guilford Press.

Gillam, J. E. (2003). Targeted prevention is not enough. *Prevention and Treatment, 6*, 196-204.

Gilligan, C. (1993). *In a different voice: Psychological theory and women's development.* Cambridge, MA: Harvard University Press.

Gordon, B., & Allen. J. (1990). Helping men in couple relationships. In R. L. Meth, R. S. Pasick, B. Gordon, J. A. Allen, L. B. Feldman, & S. Gordon (Eds.), *Men in therapy: The challenge of change* (pp. 181-208). New York, NY: Guilford Press.

Gotlib, I. H., Lewinsohn, P. M., & Seeley, J. R. (1995). Symptoms versus a diagnosis of depression: Differences in psychosocial functioning. *Journal of Consulting and Clinical Psychology, 63*, 90-100.

Harvey, V. (1999). Young women and their struggle to balance autonomy and affiliation. In M. B. Nadien & F. L. Denmark (Eds.), *Females and autonomy: A lifespan perspective.* (pp. 73-100). Boston: Allyn and Bacon.

Jack, D. C. (1991). *Silencing the self: Women and depression.* Cambridge, MA: Harvard University Press.

Jack, D. C. (1999). Silencing the self: Inner dialogues and outer realities. In T. Joiner & J. C. Coyne (Eds.), *The interactional nature of depression: Advances in interpersonal approaches* (pp. 221-246). Washington, DC: American Psychological Association.

Jack, D. C., & Dill, D. (1992). The Silencing the Self Scale: Schemas of intimacy associated with depression in women. *Psychology of Women Quarterly, 16*, 97-106.

Kaplan, A. G. (1986). The "self-in-relation": Implications for depression in women. *Psychotherapy: Theory, Research, Practice, Training, 23*, 234-242.

Kelly, A. E., & Achter, J. A. (1995). Self-concealment and attitudes toward counseling in university students. *Journal of Counseling Psychology, 42*, 40-46.

Kessler, R. C., McGonagle, K. A., Zhou, S., Nelson, C. B., Hughes, M., Eshleman, S., Wittchen, H. U., & Kendler, K. S. (1994). Lifetime and 12-month prevalence of DSM-III-R psychiatric disorders in the United States: Results from the National Comorbidity Survey. *Archives of General Psychiatry, 51*, 8-19.

Kopper, B. A., & Epperson, D. L. (1996). The experience and expression of anger: Relationships with gender, gender role socialization, depression, and mental health functioning. *Journal of Counseling Psychology, 43*, 158-165.

Le, H. N., MuZoz, R. F., Ippen, C. G., & Stoddard, J. L. (2003). Treatment is not enough: We must prevent major depression in women. *Prevention and Treatment, 6*, 289-303.

Nolen-Hoeksema, S. (1995). Epidemiology and theories of gender differences in unipolar depression. In M. V. Seeman (Ed.), *Gender and psychopathology* (pp. 63-87). Washington, DC: American Psychiatric Press.

Page, J. R., Stevens, H. B., & Galvin, S. L. (1996). Relationships between depression, self-esteem, and self-silencing behavior. *Journal of Social and Clinical Psychology*, *15*, 381-396.

Parks, A. C., & Herman, K. C. (2003). A sociocultural perspective on the primary prevention of depression. *Prevention and Treatment*, *6*, 183-204.

Rollins, J. (1996). *Women's minds, women's bodies: The psychology of women in a biosocial context*. Upper Saddle River, NJ: Prentice Hall.

Smolak, L., & Munstertieger, B. F. (2002). The relationship of gender and voice to depression and eating disorders. *Psychology of Women Quarterly*, *26*, 234-241.

Spielberger, C. D. (1999). *State-Trait Anger Expression Inventory-2*. Lutz, FL: Psychological Assessment Resources, Inc.

Thompson, J. (1995). Silencing the self: Depressive symptomatology and close relationships. *Psychology of Women Quarterly*, *19*, 337-353.

Thompson, J. M., Whiffen, V. E., & Aube, J. A. (2001). Does self-silencing link perceptions of care from parents and partners with depressive symptoms? *Journal of Social and Personal Relationships*, *18*, 503-516.

Willis-Brandon, C. (1989). *Eat like a lady: Guide for overcoming bulimia*. Deerfield Beach, FL: Health Communications, Inc.

Motivational Orientation, Expectancies, and Vulnerability for Depression in Women

Peter Horvath, PhD
Glyn Bissix, PhD
John Sumarah, PhD
Erin Crouchman, BA
Jennifer Bowdrey, BSc

INTRODUCTION

Beck's (1983) congruence theory of depression proposed that two personal styles, sociotropy and autonomy, predispose individuals for depression. The sociotropic individual is dependent, values social relations, and seeks approval from others. Individuals high on autonomy value independence and control and show perfectionism. Sociotropic and autonomous individuals are thought to be sensitive to failure experiences in their particular valued areas, for example, in relationships and achievement, respectively. However, research findings testing the congruence theory of depression have been inconsistent, with more support found for the effects of matching stress on sociotropy than autonomy (Clark, Beck, & Brown, 1992; Mazure, Bruce, Maciejewski, & Jacobs, 2000). These findings suggest that the role of personality vulnerabilities in depression needs further examination and clarification.

Recently, it has been suggested that further understanding of these personal styles as vulnerabilities for mood disorders rests on understanding the factors themselves independent of their conjunction to life events (Santor, 2003). Beck's (1983) original descriptions of these personal styles suggested motivational and coping components. Campbell and Kwon (2001) conceptualized these personal styles in motivational terms as goal-directed strategies to attain self-worth. The purpose of the present study was to examine possible motivational components that may account for the vulnerabilities in these personal styles.

Motivation and Depression

Vulnerability for depression may be based on instability in self-worth and inadequate means for regulating it. For example, Champion and Power (1995) have proposed that depression-prone individuals are ambivalent about their self-worth and have a limited set of goals that they can use to secure their sense of purpose and self-esteem. If these goals are thwarted, it is difficult to protect their self-esteem because few other goals or sources of satisfaction can be substituted for them. Fragile self-esteem and difficulties in regulating it have been linked to experiencing depression (Roberts & Monroe, 1999). Discrepancies between an individual's perceptions of ideal self and actual self-states have been associated with experiencing depression (Moretti, Rein, & Wiebe, 1998). Sociotropy and autonomy have been associated with actual-ideal self-discrepancies (Fairbrother & Moretti, 1998).

Dykman's (1998) motivational approach proposes that depression vulnerability has its origins in concerns to validate one's self-worth. Validation-seeking individuals are insecure and are preoccupied with proving themselves. How motivational orientations predispose one to depression may be further elucidated by considering the relationship of intrinsic and extrinsic motives to satisfaction and well-being, as proposed in self-determination theory (Ryan & Deci, 2000). In inclinations toward mastery and spontaneous interest in things, as found in intrinsic motivation, the locus of self-determination is internal or under the control of the person. In extrinsic motivation, in contrast, the goals and the locus of self-determination are based on standards that feel externally imposed. Extrinsic motives are dependent on outcomes that are often uncertain, and may ultimately lead to dissatisfaction, alienation, and depression. Validation-seeking individuals show a similar preoccupation with externally-based outcomes to prove their self-worth.

Santor (2003) suggested that sociotropic and autonomous individuals are trying to meet basic needs for sociability and self-worth. The preoccupation with proving one's self-worth, as seen in validation seeking, may be an active component that fosters vulnerability for depression in sociotropy and autonomy. The manner of achieving this might differ, however, with the focus on seeking social approval in sociotropy and on seeking achievement in autonomy. Furthermore, if the external approval or expectations are not met, then the individual with these personal styles might be further distressed and disappointed.

Expectancies, Social Context, and Depression

Expectancies have also been linked to depression. They have been shown to mediate the effects of self-attributions for failures on depression, as outlined in the hopelessness theory of depression (Tripp, Catano, & Sullivan, 1997). The contributions of expectancies to the onset of dysphoria or depressive symptoms in sociotropic and autonomous individuals have been recently examined by Campbell and Kwon (2001). They found that both personal styles and domain-specific hope (interpersonal and achievement oriented) made unique contributions to the prediction of dysphoria in both men and women. An interaction between personal styles and hope in predicting dysphoria was also found among women. The level of domain-specific hope with regard to meeting autonomous and sociotropic goals moderated the effects of personal styles on dysphoria. Both high achievement and interpersonal hope acted as protective factors to lower dysphoria among women high on autonomy.

These findings are consistent with the view that the social context and gender role stereotypes are important factors in the genesis of dysphoria (Mazure, Keita, & Blehar, 2002). Women are in a more vulnerable situation than men because their opportunities for achievement are more limited. Women focusing on achievement are in a doubly vulnerable position because of fewer opportunities for achievement than men but with the demands on them to fulfill social roles still remaining. However, interpersonal hope or achievement expectations appear to protect them against depression.

Women and Depression

Disadvantages in socioeconomic conditions and the limiting social roles, expectations, and demands that women face, and often adopt, result in their disempowerment and discouragement (Scattolon & Stoppard, 1999; Stoppard, 1999). Feminist authors have also pointed out that the motivational and coping orientations of women make them vulnerable to depression. There are social pressures and expectation on women to place the needs of others ahead of their own desires and to "silence the self" (Jack, 1999). Women are concerned that failing to meet others' expectations or standards will result in their rejection (Moretti et al., 1998). These extrinsic expectations and motivational orientations make them more vulnerable to depression than men.

The Present Study

If sociotropy and autonomy personal styles involve precarious motivational and coping orientations to meet unfulfilled needs for self-worth through social approval and achievement seeking, respectively, then they may lead to chronic insecurities, dissatisfactions, and subclinical levels of depression in women. Furthermore, their impact on the onset of depression would also depend on whether the goals sought are perceived to be (or expected) to be met. Therefore, the association of personal styles with depression would be moderated by outcome appraisals or expectations. If desires for self-worth through social acceptance or personal competence are perceived as not likely to be met, then an increase in depression would likely occur. Expectations of the self (e.g., self-efficacy) or perception of one's circumstances (e.g., social support) would interact with autonomy and sociotropy to determine dysphoria or depression.

The present research attempted to clarify the contributions of motivational orientations and expectancies with regard to the association of personality vulnerabilities with depressive symptoms in a community sample of women. Employing a community or a normal sample is an appropriate way to examine the effects of pre-morbid vulnerability factors on the onset of depression (Dykman, 1998). We proposed that validation seeking, as a motivational factor, would mediate the association between both sociotropy and autonomy and depressive symptoms. Secondly, we predicted that the association of sociotropy and autonomy with depressive symptoms would be moderated by expectations and perceptions of how likely social and achievement needs would be met. Individuals high on sociotropy and autonomy would be at greater risk to develop depressive symptoms when they also have negative expectancies and perceptions. Therefore, we also hypothesized that personal and social expectations would interact with autonomy and sociotropy to predict depressive symptoms in women.

METHOD

Procedure

We surveyed women residents from six communities in Kings County, Nova Scotia. Women who had reached the age of majority in the province (19 years of age or above) were selected randomly from the telephone directory. Those who agreed to participate were sent a package of questionnaires and were asked to return them by mail. The package contained consent forms and questionnaires on sociotropy and autonomy, validation-seeking goal orientations, perceived social support and expectancies, as well as demographic variables. A total of 2,297 women were called. Of this group 599 consented to participate and were sent the survey in the mail. A total of 299 surveys were returned (50%), of which 284 were complete and usable (47.4%).

Participants

On average, the sample of 284 women was middle aged (*M* = 48.50, *SD* = 16.86). The largest segments of the sample were married (66.2%), with two children (*M* = 2.24, *SD* = 1.65), homemakers (33.1% homemakers; 21.6% full-time employed), with some college education (23.9%), white (86.6% Caucasian), with a middle class family income (18.0% $30,000-39,000 Can). They lived in a small town (28.2% 1,000-2,900 population size), had half a dozen close friends (*M* = 5.63, *SD* = 4.05), were satisfied in their relationship (*M* = 8.29, *SD* = 2.13) and satisfied with their friendships (*M* = 8.19, *SD* = 1.98). The overall depression score of the sample (*M* = 11.30, *SD* = 10.32) was below the cut-off score for depression and only slightly higher than the means of the original community derivation samples used to develop the CES-D depression scale.

Measures

Demographic Questions. Data was obtained on gender, age, relationship status, number of children, number of close friends, relationship satisfaction (rated 1-10), friendship satisfaction level (rated 1-10), employment status, socioeconomic status, education, ethnic background, and local population size.

Centre for Epidemiological Studies–Depression (CES-D; Radloff, 1977). The CES-D is a 20-item self-report measure of depressive symptoms in untreated community samples. Individuals rate each item on a scale from 0 (rarely or none of the time) to 3 (most of the time) as to how often, during the past week, they have experienced various depressive symptoms. A cut off score of 16 or over is used to indicate depression. The Cronbach coefficient alpha for the CES-D in the present sample was .91.

Personal Style Inventory (PSI; Robins et al., 1994). The PSI is a 48-item self-report measure of two personal styles, sociotropy and autonomy, thought to be vulnerabilities for depression. Each item is rated on a scale from 1 (strongly disagree) to 6 (strongly agree). The sociotropy scale has 24 items measuring concerns about interpersonal relations and consists of three subscales: concerns about what others think (e.g., "I am very sensitive to criticism by others"), dependency (e.g., "I find it difficult to be alone all day"), and pleasing others (e.g., "I often put other people's needs before my own"). The autonomy scale has 24 items measuring concerns about achievement, control, and independence in three subscales: perfectionism/self-criticism (e.g., "It bothers me when I feel that I am only average and ordinary"), need for control (e.g., "I resent it when people try to direct my behavior or activities"), and defensive separation (e.g., "I tend to keep other people at a distance"). Alpha coefficients of .89 for sociotropy and .87 for autonomy were obtained in the present study.

Goal Orientation Inventory (GOI; Dykman, 1998). The GOI is a 36-item self-report measure of goal orientation. Each item is rated on a scale from 1 (strongly disagree) to 7 (strongly agree). The GOI consists of two subscales: validation-seeking (VS) orientation and growth-seeking (GS) orientation. Only the effects of validation seeking are reported in this study. Validation-seeking individuals have a strong need to establish or prove their basic worth, competence, or likeability. An example of a validation-seeking item is, "Instead of just enjoying activities and social interactions, most situations to me feel like a major test of my basic worth, competence, or likeability." Depressive symptoms were found to be associated with validation seeking (Dykman, 1998). The alpha coefficient for the validation-seeking scale used in the present sample was .96.

Social Hopelessness Scale (SHO; Flett & Hewitt, 2001). This is a 20-item self-report scale of people's perceptions and expectations about their interpersonal relations and social world. It measures negative perception and expectations for interpersonal themes such as the type and availability of relationships, exposure to mistreatment and criticism, lack of support, negative social comparisons, and hopelessness about social situations and relationships. A 5-point Likert scale is used to rate items from 1 (strongly disagree) to 5 (strongly agree). Sample items include "I expect that some people will always be mean to me" and "It is impossible for me to avoid being hurt by others." An alpha coefficient of .88 was obtained in the present sample.

Sense of Support Scale (SSS; Dolbier & Steinhardt, 2000). The SSS is a 21-item measure of perceived social support. Participants rate each statement on a 4-point Likert scale ranging from 0 (not at all true) to 3 (completely true). The scale consists of items that measure the perceived quality of social support. Sample items include "I have friendships that are mutually fulfilling" and "I feel well supported by my friends and/or family." Six of the items are reverse scored. A coefficient alpha of .88 was found in the present sample.

The General Self-Efficacy Scale (GSE; Sherer et al., 1982). The GSE is a 17-item subscale taken from the Self-Efficacy Scale measuring self-perceptions of initiating, sustaining effort, and persisting in aversive conditions. Each item is scored from 1 (strongly disagree) to 14 (strongly agree). Ten of the items are reverse scored. Sample items include, "I feel secure about my ability to do things" and "When unexpected problems occur, I don't handle them well." The alpha in the present sample was .89.

RESULTS

Motivational Aspects of Personal Styles in Predicting Depressive Symptoms

Hierarchical regressions were used to test the hypothesis that validation-seeking goal orientation mediates the relationship between personal styles and depression. To demonstrate this mediation effect in the present study, the following criteria had to be met (Baron & Kenny, 1986): (i) the personal style needed to be significantly associated with depressive symptoms; (ii) validation-seeking goal orientation needed to be significantly associated with personal style; (iii) validation-seeking needed to be significantly related to depressive symptoms, and (iv) when personal style and validation-seeking were entered simultaneously into a multiple regression equation predicting depressive symptoms, the partial correlation between personal style and depressive symptoms needed to be smaller than their zero-order correlation. Consistent with criterion (i), the two personal styles were significantly correlated with depressive symptoms (sociotropy $r = .42, p < .001$; autonomy $r = .45, p < .001$). Consistent with criterion (ii), validation-seeking was significantly correlated with sociotropy ($r = .64, p < .001$) and autonomy ($r = .61, p < .001$). Consistent with criterion (iii), validation-seeking was significantly correlated with depressive symptoms ($r = .53, p < .001$).

To further test the mediation hypothesis, depressive symptoms were regressed on personal styles and validation seeking separately for sociotropy and autonomy. Consistent with criterion iv), when sociotropy and validation seeking were both in the regression equation [$R^2 = .34, F(2, 210) = 54.09, p < .001$], the partial correlation between sociotropy and depressive symptoms was no longer significant, $pr = .07$, ns. Similarly, when autonomy and validation-seeking were both in the regression equation

[$R^2 = .28, F(2, 210) = 41.04, p < .001$], the partial correlation showed that the association between autonomy and depressive symptoms was reduced considerably ($pr = .17, p < .05$). Thus, our findings indicated that sociotropy and autonomy increased the risk for depressive symptoms through the mediating influence of validation-seeking goal orientation.

Expectancies as Moderators of the Effects of Personal Styles on Depressive Symptoms

We tested the hypothesis that expectancies and perceptions moderate the relationship between personality styles and depressive symptoms. Consistent with Baron and Kenny's (1986) recommendation, moderator effects were tested with hierarchical multiple regressions predicting depressive symptoms. First, the personality variable was entered into the regression equation, followed by the expectancy variable, and finally by the interaction between the personality and the expectancy variables.

Separate analyses were conducted for sociotropy and autonomy. First, we tested the hypothesis that social hopelessness moderates the association between sociotropy and depression (see Table 1). Both sociotropy and social hopelessness predicted depressive symptoms. The interaction term between sociotropy and social hopelessness was also significant. Similar findings were obtained for autonomy.

Next, we tested the hypothesis that perception of social support moderates the association between sociotropy and depressive symptoms (see Table 2). Both sociotropy and perceived social support predicted depressive symptoms. The interaction term between sociotropy and perceived

TABLE 1. Hierarchical Multiple Regressions Predicting Depressive Symptoms from Personal Styles and Social Hopelessness

	Sociotropy				Autonomy			
	r	*pr*	ΔR^2	*F*	*r*	*pr*	ΔR^2	*F*
Personality	.42***	.25***	.17	44.24***	.45***	.22**	.20	49.14***
SH	.57***	.47 ***	.19	64.24***	.57***	.39***	.14	42.74***
Interaction	.21**	.14*	.01	3.90*	.27***	.17*	.02	5.71*

Notes: SH = Social Hopelessness; *F*-value is associated with the change in R^2. *r* = zero order correlation with depressive symptoms; *pr* = partial correlation with depressive symptoms; ΔR^2 = change in R^2 when variable entered into equation.

social support was also significant. Similar findings were obtained for autonomy.

Next, we tested the hypothesis that the perception of self-efficacy moderates the association between sociotropy and depressive symptoms (see Table 3). Both sociotropy and perceived self-efficacy predicted depressive symptoms. The interaction term between sociotropy and perceived self-efficacy was also significant. Similar main effects were obtained for autonomy. The interaction term between autonomy and perceived self-efficacy showed a trend similar to those mentioned above but was not significant.

The significant interaction terms were explored further to determine the source of the interactions. High and low levels of the interacting variables

TABLE 2. Hierarchical Multiple Regressions Predicting Depressive Symptoms from Personal Styles and Perceived Social Support

	Sociotropy				Autonomy			
	r	*pr*	ΔR^2	*F*	*r*	*pr*	ΔR^2	*F*
Personality	.42***	.42***	.17	39.98***	.45***	.33***	.21	53.33***
SS	–.51***	–.53***	.24	78.27***	–.51***	–.39***	.14	41.29***
Interaction	–.22**	–.19**	.02	7.13**	–.33***	–.22**	.03	9.74**

Notes: SS = Social Support; *F*-value is associated with the change in R^2. r = zero order correlation with depressive symptoms; *pr* = partial correlation with depressive symptoms; ΔR^2 = change in R^2 when variable entered into equation.
*$p < .05$; **$p < .01$; ***$p < .001$.

TABLE 3. Hierarchical Multiple Regressions Predicting Depressive Symptoms from Personal Styles and Perceived Self-Efficacy

	Sociotropy				Autonomy			
	r	*pr*	ΔR^2	*F*	*r*	*pr*	ΔR^2	*F*
Personality	.42***	.33***	.18	49.81***	.45***	.36***	.20	55.43***
GSE	–.52***	–.45***	.18	63.09***	–.52***	–.43***	.15	52.73***
Interaction	–.15**	–.14*	.01	4.49**	–.15*	–.11^t	.01	2.77^t

Notes: GSE = General Self-Efficacy; *F*-value is associated with the change in R^2. r = zero order correlation with depressive symptoms; *pr* = partial correlation with depressive symptoms; ΔR^2 = change in R^2 when variable entered into equation.
$^t p < .10$; * $p < .05$; ** $p < .01$; *** $p < .001$.

were estimated by calculating their mean and by adding or subtracting the value for 1 standard deviation (Cohen & Cohen, 1983). These values were then substituted into the regression equation, which was then used to predict depression scores at all possible combinations of high and low levels of the interacting variables. Examination of the plots of the interactions between sociotropy and expectancies showed that as sociotropy increased, the effects of high social hopelessness on depressive symptoms also increased. Similarly, as autonomy increased, the effects of high social hopelessness on depressive symptoms also increased. Similar configurations were found for the interactions between these two personal styles and perceived low social support and low self-efficacy.

DISCUSSION

Our findings help to clarify the nature of the vulnerability for depression present in personal styles. The association of sociotropy and autonomy with depressive symptoms appears to be mediated, at least in part, by validation-seeking goal orientations. The desire to acquire self-worth through obtaining external approval appears to be a major component in the vulnerability for dysphoria. Research has shown that such externally-focused motives are negatively associated with long-term satisfaction and well-being (Ryan & Deci, 2000). Attempts to acquire self-worth through meeting external goals or standards are precarious and unpredictable. These motivational orientations likely make the individual frustrated, dissatisfied, and vulnerable to disappointment. Subclinical forms of depression or dysphoria are likely to be present in personal styles based on such motivational orientations. If the external validation that the person is seeking appears as not likely to be met, then the individual may become further disappointed and even more susceptible for depression.

The motivational approach we have taken is consistent with the recognized importance of situational factors in the development of depression in women (Mazure et al., 2002). Some forms of motivation and coping are less adaptive in certain environments than in others. When the environment changes and becomes less supportive, the outcome-based orientations to acquire self-worth present in sociotropy and autonomy can turn out to be unsuccessful. Therefore, negative outcomes and expectations can result in despondency. Feminist theories of depression have also emphasized the importance of environmental or contextual factors in the onset of depression in women (Scattolon & Stoppard, 1999; Stoppard, 1999). Women have fewer opportunities in society and face pressures to adopt social roles and personal styles that expose them to the vagaries of external circumstances that impact on their self-worth. If the individual accepts that her self-worth is contingent on the occurrence of certain external events, they place themselves at increased risk. By losing control over evaluation of their self-worth, individuals may find themselves highly vulnerable to the effects of circumstances. Community interventions and public education will need to teach and encourage women not to succumb to social pressures that would deprive them of control over the evaluation of their self-worth. Psychological interventions could also attempt to change individuals' externally-oriented frames of reference used to make attributions of self-worth.

Although our study did not test a clinical sample, it has been argued that research based on subclinical levels of depression and dysphoria can help to clarify the processes involved in depression more generally (Campbell & Kwon, 2001; Dykman, 1998). Our approach is compatible with this proposal. The precursors of clinical depression may be dysphoria or subclinical levels of depression that are independent of specific events (Dykman, 1998). However, as our study has shown, these low moods can be exacerbated by negative expectations or environmental outcomes. Under such circumstances vulnerable individuals may develop more severe forms of depression. It is also possible that the vulnerability is due to the fact that individuals with these personal styles do not make good use of ego defenses that could protect their self-esteem from negative outcomes. Research will need to further examine such motivational, coping, and defensive processes that may contribute to the vulnerability in these personal styles.

REFERENCES

Baron, R. M., & Kenny, D. A. (1986). The moderator-mediator variable distinction in social psychological research: Conceptual, strategic, and statistical considerations. *Journal of Personality and Social Psychology, 51*, 1173-1182.

Beck, A. T. (1983). Cognitive therapy of depression: New perspectives. In P. J. Clayton & J. E. Barrett (Eds.). *Treatment of depression: Old controversies and new approaches* (pp. 265-290). New York: Raven.

Campbell, D. G., & Kwon, P. (2001). Domain-specific hope and personal style: Toward an integrative understanding of dysphoria. *Journal of Social and Clinical Psychology, 20*, 498-520.

Champion, L. A., & Power, M. J. (1995). Social and cognitive approaches to depression: Towards a new synthesis. *British Journal of Clinical Psychology, 34*, 485-503.

Clark, D. A., Beck, A. T., & Brown, G. K. (1992). Sociotropy, autonomy, and life event perceptions in dysphoric and nondysphoric individuals. *Cognitive Therapy and Research, 16*, 635-652.

Cohen, J., & Cohen, P. (1983). *Applied multiple regression/correlational analysis for the behavioral sciences* (2nd ed.). Hillsdale, NJ: Lawrence Erlbaum.

Dolbier, C. L., & Steinhardt, M. A. (2000). The development and validation of the Sense of Support Scale. *Behavioral Medicine*, *25*, 169-179.

Dykman, B. M. (1998). Integrating cognitive and motivational factors in depression: Initial tests of a goal-orientation approach. *Journal of Personality and Social Psychology*, *74*, 139-158.

Fairbrother, N., & Moretti, M. (1998). Sociotropy, autonomy, and self-discrepancy: Status in depressed, remitted depressed, and control participants. *Cognitive Therapy and Research*, *22*, 279-296.

Flett, G. L., & Hewitt, P. L. (2001, June 23). *Social hopelessness and personality factors in depression.* Paper presented at the annual convention of the Canadian Psychological Association, Laval University, Ste-Foy, Quebec.

Jack, D. C. (1999). Silencing the self: Inner dialogues and outer realities. In T. Joiner & J. C. Coyne (Eds.), *The interactional nature of depression: Advances in interpersonal approaches* (pp. 221-246). Washington, DC: American Psychological Association.

Mazure, C. M., Bruce, M. L., Maciejewski, P. K., & Jacobs, S. C. (2000). Adverse life events and cognitive-personality characteristics in the prediction of major depression and antidepressant response. *American Journal of Psychiatry*, *157*, 869-903.

Mazure, C. M., Keita, G. P., & Blehar, M. C. (2002). *Summit on women and depression: Proceedings and recommendations.* Washington, DC: American Psychological Association. Available at: http://www.apa.org/pi/wpo/women&depression.pdf.

Moretti, M. M., Rein, A. S., & Wiebe, V. J. (1998). Relational self-regulation: Gender differences in risk for dysphoria. *Canadian Journal of Behavioural Science*, *30*, 243-252.

Radloff, L. S. (1977). The CES-D scale: A self-report depression scale for research in the general population. *Applied Psychological Measurement*, *1*, 385-401.

Roberts, J. E., & Monroe, S. M. (1999). Vulnerable self-esteem and social processes in depression: Toward an interpersonal model of self-esteem regulation. In T. Joiner & J. C. Coyne (Eds.), *The interactional nature of depression: Advances in interpersonal approaches* (pp. 149-187). Washington, DC: American Psychological Association.

Robins, C. J., Ladd, J., Welkowitz, J., Blaney, P. H., Diaz, R., & Kutcher, G. (1994). The Personal Style Inventory: Preliminary validation studies of new measures of sociotropy and autonomy. *Journal of Psychopathology and Behavioral Assessment*, *16*, 277-300.

Ryan, R. M., & Deci, E. L. (2000). Self-determination theory and the facilitation of intrinsic motivation, social development, and well-being. *American Psychologist*, *55*, 68-78.

Santor, D. (2003). Proximal effects of dependency and self-criticism: Conceptual and methodological challenges for depressive vulnerability research. *Cognitive Behaviour Therapy*, *32*, 49-67.

Scattolon, Y., & Stoppard, J. M. (1999). "Getting on with life": Women's experiences and ways of coping with depression. *Canadian Psychology*, *40*, 205-219.

Sherer, M., Maddux, J. E., Mercandante, B., Prentice-Dunn, S., Jacobs, B., & Rogers, R. W. (1982). The Self-Efficacy Scale: Construction and validation. *Psychological Reports*, *51*, 663-671.

Stoppard, J. M. (1999). Why new perspectives are needed for understanding depression in women. *Canadian Psychology*, *40*, 79-90.

Tripp, D. A., Catano, V., & Sullivan, M. J. L. (1997). The contributions of attributional style, expectancies, depression, and self-esteem in a cognition-based depression model. *Canadian Journal of Behavioural Science*, *29*, 101-111.

Exploring Perceptions of Alcohol Use as Self-Medication for Depression Among Women Receiving Community-Based Treatment for Alcohol Problems

Catrina G. Brown, PhD
Sherry H. Stewart, PhD

INTRODUCTION

While extant literature reports a co-existence between alcohol use and depression among women, the dynamics of this relationship requires further exploration (e.g., Abraham & Fava, 1999; Grant & Hartford, 1995).[1] It has been consistently demonstrated that women are more likely than men to have a co-occurring problem with alcohol use and depression (Hartka et al., 1991; Helzer & Pryzbeck, 1988). Women are more likely than men to drink in response to depression (Helzer & Pryzbeck, 1988) and are more likely to use alcohol in response to both severe (Gilman & Abraham, 2001) and less severe (Weiss, Griffin, & Tobin, 1992) depression than men. Thus, women appear to self-medicate across a range of depression symptom severity including dysthymia, revealing an increased risk of alcohol abuse problems across the depression severity continuum (Kocsis, Markowitz, & Prien, 1990). Some researchers have claimed that depression is the result of chronic alcohol abuse rather than the cause (e.g., Schuckit et al., 1997). However, important often unacknowledged gender differences have emerged about patterns of this relationship. In particular, depression appears to most often follow alcohol abuse in men, but to most often precede it for women (e.g., Gilman & Abraham, 2001; Kessler et al., 1997). Among women sampled in the Epidemiologic Catchment Area study 66% reported depression preceding alcohol use (Hodgins, el-Guebably, Armstrong, & Dufour, 1999), whereas 78% of men reported that alcohol dependence preceded the onset of depression.

These gender differences suggests the possibility that women may use alcohol to self-medicate for depression. Self-medication with alcohol can be understood as a method to reduce or manage emotional pain and suffering (Khantzian, 1990). The social context of women's depression and alcohol use, including social histories of trauma and abuse (e.g., Jarvis & Copeland, 1997; Stewart & Israeli, 2003; Stoppard, 1999), lends support to the notion that women use alcohol as a form of self-medication for depression.

In the present investigation, we explored women's experiences of depression and alcohol use problems, and the underlying mechanisms of this association.[2] We focus here on data which emerged from qualitative interviews on the relations of depression and alcohol use and seek to gain a better understanding of: (1) women's experiences of the relationship between depression and alcohol use problems, (2) the extent to which women use alcohol as a form of self-medicating for depression including relief and reward drinking, and (3) the gendered social context of these experiences.[3] This paper explores the meanings that women with alcohol problems attach to their experiences of the relationship between their depression and their use of alcohol.

METHOD

Participants

Fifty-eight adult women (aged 18 years or older) seeking treatment for alcohol abuse or dependence were recruited through Addiction Prevention and Treatment Services (Capital District Health) in Halifax, Nova Scotia for the larger study of which this investigation is a part (see Note 3). All of the women who self-identified as problem drinkers by appearing for the study met criteria for a likely alcohol use disorder on the alcoholism screening test (i.e., score of 6 or higher on the Brief Michigan Alcoholism Screening Test; Pokorny, Miller, & Kaplan, 1972). Eighteen women agreed to participate in open-ended semi-structured taped interviews and were later contacted and scheduled for interviews. The mean age of the 18 women participating in the open-ended interviews was 38 years of age. Women interviewed had an average education level of 14 years. Limited income and unemployment was a concern for 13 of the 18 women.

Procedures

Willing and eligible women who were participating in the larger questionnaire-based study (Stewart et al., 2006) were scheduled for a later qualitative interview. Data was gathered on self-reported experiences of depression and co-existing alcohol use problems through in-depth semi-structured qualitative interviews of 18 women. We did not use standardized measures of depression as the theme of depression emerged during qualitative interviews in the larger study on the relationship between binge eating and heavy drinking, and it was not an *a priori* purpose of the larger study to investigate relations of depression and alcohol misuse. Women's self-reporting of depression included a history of their depression, and use of prescribed anti-depressants. Two hour-long audio taped interviews emphasized women's experiences of their alcohol use. In this paper we report on the portion of the research that centers on women's perceptions of the relationship between depression and alcohol use as self-medication. Pseudonyms were chosen by each of the women interviewed and used in the presentation of findings rather than real names.

Data Analysis

Analysis identified dominant themes and narratives that emerged with respect to women's alcohol use as self-medication for depression. Those themes that were most salient and most frequent were identified. The data analysis involved overlapping thematic analysis. We began with open coding to generate categories. We then coded for connections between identified categories, and finally used selective coding to integrate the categories through uncovering the dominant story, or "explicating the story line" in the stories told (Strauss & Corbin, 1990, p.119). A thematic analysis of the data involved "a search for and identification of common threads that extend throughout an entire interview or set of interviews" (Morse & Field, 1995, p.139). This strategy allowed us to unpack, contextualize, and interpret the narratives that emerged in this study.

RESULTS

Interview findings of experiences and perceptions of alcohol use as self-medication for depression among women in community-based treatment for alcohol use problems is reported here. We found that all 18 women interviewed reported life-time histories of depression. Moreover, 14 of the 18 (78%) women interviewed reported currently using anti-depressant medication, although they were not queried as to the nature of the conditions for which they were prescribed the antidepressants (e.g., depressive disorder, anxiety disorder, eating disorder).

Thematic analyses of women's descriptions of their reasons for drinking showed that alcohol was used by women to self-medicate for depression by relieving painful emotional experiences (reported by all 18 women) and by producing a sense of pleasure (reported by 15 of the 18 women) (Stewart et al., 2006). Drinking to relieve painful emotional experiences provided women with a means of escape, numbing them from overwhelmingly painful emotions that they often felt powerless to change. Descriptions of drinking to produce pleasure suggested that this form of drinking provided women with greater self-confidence, and increased their capacity to have fun. Additionally, it was frequently reported that when they were drinking, women felt more confident and comfortable in social situations, especially in relating to men. Overall, while both types of drinking were reported as a way to self-medicate for experiences of depression (e.g., reward drinking provided opportunities for pleasure that were otherwise missing in their lives), relief drinking was a more predominant theme.

Women's Experience of the Relationship Between Depression and Alcohol Use

Women's stories consistently convey overwhelming dissatisfaction with themselves and their lives. Descriptions of depression are characterized by a profound sense of hopelessness, powerlessness, deprivation, lack of emotional and financial resources, isolation and self-contempt. Life seems to present endless obstacles which women often feel unable to maneuver. Further, women seem to believe life has passed them by, and that they can not expect it to offer them much. Women describe the relationship between depression and use of alcohol in their lives:

> My life has been so horrible. I must have been cursed when I was born. These were feelings and thoughts that I had. Life has always been so difficult and so bad and so traumatic that I never honestly believed it was ever going to get any better. So I might as well drink/use. . . . You're a loser, you always will be. . . . I've heard other people describe it the same way, like this black hole that you fall into. There's just no way out. (Charlotte)

> If I had something to drink, I wouldn't feel so rotten. And this happened a lot. . . . I was generally very depressed. So I used alcohol to lessen the depression. But then when I decide not to, then I had to deal with the depression because there it was. I couldn't get away from it. . . . I had major depression most of my life. I had very short periods of feeling good. . . . maybe a few months. The rest of the time I was very depressed. (Molly)

All of the women report using alcohol as a way to regulate emotional states and report experiencing depression prior to alcohol use; however, some also note that depression is exacerbated by alcohol use. While women often report feeling badly or depressed after drinking, they attribute this to intense self-criticism for having "lost control," in addition to the negative consequences of drinking on their life (e.g., losing their children, continued poverty and unemployment, relationship breakdown, negative impact on family life, and greater risk for physical and sexual violence). Despite these longer-term negative consequences, drinking offers ways to cope and self-medicate in the short term.

Drinking as Self-Medication

Women report seeking to escape or find solace from painful emotional realities. Numbing oneself through alcohol use is frequently described as a coping mechanism:

> . . . numb is good. You don't feel when you're numb. You don't think when you're numb. And you don't have to experience anything when you're numb. And sometimes it's the only way you can go through life. (Shelley)

Most women report a need to escape from their lives. Binge drinking self-medicates by providing this sense of escape:

> . . . to kill the pain, and to hide from the world. . . . I just used to drink until I felt okay. . . . I drank to kill the pain and the hurt of the marriage that I was in (Chelsea)

In addition to drinking to relieve negative emotions, some women report the use of drinking as a form of emotional reward. Even this second type of drinking can be seen in the light of self-medicating for depression as it provides women with some of the positive emotions that are otherwise missing for them. In this sense they are self-medicating for the "anhedonia" or inability to experience pleasure that is often a part of the symptoms of depression.

> Sometimes I'd have a really good time. . . . I guess because I'm such a serious person it kind of lightened me up a bit. (Iris)

Drinking as self-medication can be seen, paradoxically, as a form of self-care. Most women report that they relied upon a combination of both drinking to relieve painful emotions and drinking to obtain pleasure, rather than only one or the other. Through these two types of drinking they describe a dual mechanism that provides them with both relief from emotional pain or struggle, and a way to give themselves something positive by producing a more positive mood. Charlotte believes she used alcohol to "stuff down feelings that [she] couldn't handle" and states:

> It was to create feelings of happiness and joy that I couldn't find within myself. It was to escape from any problem that life threw my way. . . . When I first started experiencing the high from drinking–it feels just great. The world has gone away. I'm protected and insulated from it. . . . The escape from life and reality. I had determined a long time ago that life was cruel. And I just couldn't handle it. (Charlotte)

> I think it's positive. It's not, because my life has been ruined because of it. But, at the time, it was what I needed. It is just like my medicine. Made me feel good. (Claire)

This dual mechanism reflects not only the need to find relief from overwhelmingly negative experiences, but to obtain alternatively, however fleeting, some form of positive experience. The craving for emotional nourishment and comfort exists within a starkly depleted emotional and social landscape.

The Context of Women's Lives and the Use of Alcohol for Self-Medication

The dual mechanism of relief and reward drinking to self-medicate for depression makes sense given the context of women's lives. The gendered context of women's self-medication stories includes a history of failed intimate relationships, irreparable loss of their children, significant childhood emotional, physical, and sexual abuse, rape and physical abuse in adulthood, and ongoing poverty. Additionally, women report that these life conditions have left them with profoundly damaged self-esteems and a lack of effective coping strategies. Ironically, most of the women's lives have actually required profound coping capacity while simultaneously robbing them of such capacity. What can be seen is that despite such difficult life circumstances these women demonstrate tremendous resilience.

A central theme in the women's stories about alcohol use and depression is the ongoing experience of difficult, painful, and abusive relationships. Women describe childhood relationships with parents that were fraught with emotional, physical and sexual abuse, only to be followed in many cases with sexual assault in adulthood, and domestic violence in their relationships with men. There is an overall sense of deprivation and lack of emotional support in relation to others. Drinking is often described as a way to deal with dissatisfaction, feelings of powerlessness, stress, and abuse in relationships, particularly their relationships with men.

> Once my husband and I started having problems, I would drink to alleviate the stress. . . . When we broke up, I used it to block out the emotional pain. (Paula)

In addition to abusive and traumatic relationships in childhood, many women report overwhelming sadness regarding the loss of their relationships with their children. Issues of mothering includes concerns about neglect, protecting their children from abuse, and struggling with trying not drinking in front of them. One woman describes the pain of giving up her son for adoption at birth when she was 18 years old.

> I walked out of that office. She [the social worker] drove me home. I went on one of the worst [drinking] binges of my life that lasted about 3 years. . . . I took anything and everything to kill absolutely every feeling that I had. (Charlotte)

Childhood violence and trauma were spontaneously reported by 16 of the 18 women interviewed for this study. Sexual abuse was spontaneously reported by 15 women, and physical abuse by 8. Multiple forms of abuse were reported by 11 of the 18 women from childhood through adulthood. Another 10 of the 18 women reported experiencing either battery from a male partner or sexual assault after adolescence. It is clear from their stories, that the women in this study had significant traumatic life experiences preceding the onset of their depression and their problematic use of alcohol. Additionally, a number of women report experiences of sexual assault while intoxicated, and physical abuse in relationships with men who also have drinking problems.

One woman was no stranger to violence in her life that she reports began when she was 4 years old. She reports: "My mother ran a whorehouse and rented her daughters. I was the youngest. . . . So the sexual abuse started at 4." She clearly connects her drinking to these painful experiences:

> It takes me out of me. I don't have to think about my childhood. I don't have to think about not working right now. I don't have to

> think about where I'm living, or if, I'm going to afford this. I don't have to worry about any of that. It takes me out of me. . . . The devil you know is better than one you don't. When you're being raped as a child, your body is being raped, but trust me, your mind is nowhere in the vicinity. I'm gone. . . . But you don't want to feel. And if you don't feel it at the time, it just stops. . . . It never goes away. You know. Until you sit down and deal with the issues that make you that way, you're never going to be able to. . . . Suicide has always been an option for me. Like I said to my counselor, drinking is not an option. Suicide is. (Shelley)

Unemployment and poverty are ongoing problems for the women in this study. Among the women participating, 13 of the 18 are unemployed with limited incomes. One woman describes her struggle with poverty and homelessness as follows:

> I had to wash my face in puddles that kind of stuff. It was dreadful. Nothing to eat. It was awful. I didn't know about food programs or anything like that. . . . I was homeless. I lived in my car. That wasn't a too happy time . . . I was starting to feel a little better when I got my own place. I felt so miserable and terrible it was just beyond belief. (Molly)

Drinking is described as a means to regulate one's internal emotional world. Feeling depressed, women often report feeling not only emotionally deprived, isolated or lonely, and craving more positive and caring relationships, but often were lacking the skills and resources to resolve these issues. Many women report difficulty acknowledging and meeting their own needs primarily because no one had ever taught them they were of any value.

> I don't know how to take care of my needs, because my needs were never taken care of. I don't have any role models. I learned how to take care of me by learning how to take care of my puppy. (Shelley)

Some women report that because of early life experiences, such as childhood sexual abuse, they never learned healthy coping strategies.

> This was my only form of escape. And anything . . . bad, sad, whatever, that happened to me. I had never learned any healthy ways to deal with life . . . I never had any healthy coping mechanisms to

> deal with anything. Anything at all. I never learned any coping mechanisms . . . because of what happened. (Charlotte)

Similarly, women suggest that negative life experiences such as childhood abuse contributes to their lack of self-worth. This lack of self-worth subsequently contributed to depression which in turn resulted in self-medication through drinking.

> It was a lot of self-esteem stuff. She used to say things like, "I wish you'd never been born." That kind of thing. So I started thinking, "I'm not a very good person. My mother doesn't love me, so I must not be much good." (Molly)

Participants report profoundly damaged views of themselves. One woman related her binge drinking to her feelings of worthlessness, and to her need to reduce emotional pain:

> I always had the little voices in my head of worthlessness . . . not having any value . . . and the alcohol takes the . . . you know, anything to soothe the pain, ease the pain. . . . And alcohol, if it didn't ease it, it just made you forget about it, at least, for a little while. . . . it just helped take the "uckiness" away. . . .You know you run to the bottle and you get it in you as fast as you can, as quick as you can, and get rid of the pain as fast and as quick as you can. . . . Trying to get rid of all that. Not have to deal with that. Just be Miss Happy. (Charlotte)

Women report that they have learned to suppress, hide or deny their emotional needs which they subsequently address through drinking. Further, women often suggest that women's addiction issues are different than men's because of the degree of shame and guilt women feel about their drinking problem.

DISCUSSION

Women in community-based treatment for alcohol problems reported that alcohol use was a form of self-medication for depression and sadness. Women used alcohol as a means of coping or self-medicating to regulate their emotional lives through relief or reward drinking. It provided relief or escape from difficult, painful, overwhelming or negative emotions.

The use of alcohol as a form of escape, to numb, or to kill emotional pain is a reoccurring theme in this research. For many, relief drinking also provides a form of comfort or self-soothing. Women also reported reward drinking as a way to produce more positive emotional states and this may be related to the anhedonia associated with depression. The simultaneous need to seek relief and reward makes sense given the overwhelming emotional pain and lack of supports and resources documented by the women in this study.

The bleak social context of these women's lives was evident in their very painful and often significantly traumatic stories. Heavy drinking appears to be a way to alleviate depression, hopelessness, and pain within their lives, especially when they feel ill equipped to contend with these experiences in any other way. While alcohol use provided the women in this study with a mechanism of temporary escape from difficult experiences, their use of alcohol produced many additional problems for them in the long run. While alcohol use was repeatedly described as a coping strategy which provided both relief and reward, it was an imperfect method in the long term, often contributing to the loss of children and other relationships, isolation, poverty and unemployment, risk of sexual assault, and, ultimately, even more severe depression. Thus, while life dissatisfaction seems to precede alcohol use problems in this study of women's experiences, alcohol use seems to almost guarantee ongoing depression and unhappiness for them. It is often suggested that one either drinks in response to depression or that depression follows alcohol use (e.g., Schuckit et al., 1997). Our findings suggest that the immediate effects of alcohol help women cope with depression, but that the long-term impact of drinking on their lives causes problems which reinforce their depression. These problems produce the ongoing need for relief or comfort, which is often met through drinking. Thus the negative consequences of drinking make the relief and reward immediately gained from drinking short lived. A vicious cycle is created when depression is worsened by drinking as it motivates further drinking in an attempt to manage the ever increasing spiral of depression.

Prevention and treatment for women with co-occurring depression and alcohol use problems needs to address childhood abuse, violence in adulthood, and poverty. Further interventions for such women need to help them develop better and more effective coping skills–ways of dealing with conflict in relationships and meeting their emotional needs. Such interventions need to assist them in developing ways to soothe and comfort themselves, to deal with overwhelming experiences of pain, failure, and loss, and to increase their sense of self-worth. When we asked women in this study about their treatment preferences, they reported the need to learn skills in self-care and coping as an alternative to use of alcohol as self-medication. Recent research on prevention suggests that when you treat such hopelessness in young people, risky drinking and drinking problems are reduced (Stewart et al., 2005). Community education on the relationship between depression and alcohol use problems could be another important aspect of prevention. Further, it is necessary to include advocacy especially in the area of child welfare, as well as assistance in obtaining needed resources (i.e., financial, child care, housing, transportation, individually-focused therapy) in women's treatment for alcohol use problems.

It is clear from this research that treatment for women's depression is likely to require simultaneous treatment for alcohol or other substance use problems, as well as trauma. Whether women seek treatment primarily for depression, or primarily for alcohol use problems, they should be screened for both, and the relationship between depression and alcohol use should be a focus when relevant within therapy. Rather than adopting a pathologizing, problem-saturated approach to depression or alcohol use, this research supports the importance of exploring what they mean to women themselves, and how they makes sense in the context of their lives. In addition, this research suggests that it would be helpful for treatment planning and setting therapy goals to explore the relationship between depression and alcohol use with women at the outset of treatment. The identification of the vicious cycle between depression and alcohol use from women's own perspectives may help encourage women to change this pattern.

There are a number of limitations of this study. As women in this study had co-occurring problems with binge eating and binge drinking, future research needs to determine whether our findings are generalizable to women with alcohol problems who don't also binge eat. This study is an initial exploratory investigation into the co-incidence of depression and alcohol use problems among women. While it provides preliminary insight into women's experience of the relationship between depression and alcohol use in their lives, future research will need to explore the mechanisms of this association further. We do not suggest that the small number of interviews in this qualitative study represents women in community-based alcohol treatment in general. However, as research on addiction often centers on men and subsequently falsely generalized to women, this study has sought to highlight women's experiences. While the findings cannot claim that men do not have similar experiences, future research would need to compare interviews between men and women. In addition, there is a need for multi-method investigations that supplement qualitative interviews on women's perceptions with quantitative measures on the relations of aspects of depressive symptoms to aspects of alcohol misuse.

NOTES

1. A high co-prevalence between depressive symptoms and disorders with alcohol problems is evident in large-scale community-based studies including the Epidemiologic Catchment Area study (ECA; Helzer & Pryzbeck, 1988), the National Co-morbidity Survey (Kessler et al., 1994), and the National Longitudinal Alcohol Epidemiological Survey (Hasin & Grant, 2002).

2. The authors would like to acknowledge the assistance of service providers and the program directors for their contribution to the project, including their assistance in providing access to the women in their treatment services and their assistance in participant recruitment. We would also like to thank Sarah Larsen and Jennifer Theakston for their research assistance. We extend our thanks to the women receiving services at these programs for their participation in the study.

3. The study reported here emerged within the context of a larger study on the relations of binge eating and heavy drinking in women receiving treatment for alcohol problems (see Stewart et al., 2006). Since the purpose of the larger study was to attempt to understand the mechanisms underlying the co-prevalence of binge eating and binge drinking among women problem drinkers, all of the women participating in the interviews had a co-existing problem of binge eating and heavy drinking. All of the women who self-identified as problem drinkers met criteria for a likely alcohol use disorder on an alcoholism screening test (i.e., score of 6 or higher on the Brief Michigan Alcoholism Screening Test). Consistent with expectations for an alcohol treatment sample the participants engaged in a pattern of frequent and heavy drinking. Further, responses to the Binge Scale (Hawkins & Clement, 1980) suggest that the vast majority of participants (90.2%) could be considered to have a "severe" problem with binge eating. The participants completed a variety of additional measures for the purposes of the larger study (see Stewart et al., 2006).

REFERENCES

Abraham, H. D., & Fava, M. (1999). Order of onset of substance abuse and depression in a sample of depressed outpatients. *Comprehensive Psychiatry*, *40*, 44-50.

Gilman, S. E., & Abraham, H. D. (2001). A longitudinal study of the order of onset of alcohol dependence and major depression. *Drug and Alcohol Dependence*, *63*, 277-286.

Grant, B. F., & Hartford, T. C. (1995). Comorbidity between DSM-IV alcohol use disorders and major depression: Results of a national survey. *Drug and Alcohol Dependence*, *39*, 197-206.

Hartka, E., Johnstone, B., Leino, V., Motoyshi, M., Temple, M., & Fillmore, K. (1991). A meta-analysis of depressive symptomatology and alcohol consumption over time. *British Journal of Addictions*, *86*, 1283-1298.

Hasin, D. S., & Grant, B. F. (2002). Major depression in 6050 former drinkers. *Archives of General Psychiatry*, *59*, 794-800.

Hawkins, R. C., & Clement, P. F. (1980). Development and construct validation of a self-report measure of binge eating tendencies. *Addictive Behaviors*, *5*, 219-226.

Helzer, J. E., & Pryzbeck, T. R. (1988). The co-occurrence of alcoholism with other psychiatric disorders in the general population and its impact on treatment. *Journal of Studies on Alcohol*, *49*, 219-224.

Hodgins, D. C., el-Guebably, N., Armstrong, S., & Dufour, M. (1999). Implications of depression outcome from alcohol dependence: A 3-year prospective follow-up. *Alcoholism: Clinical and Experimental Research*, *23*, 151-157.

Jarvis, T., & Copeland, J. (1997). Child sexual abuse as a predictor of psychiatric co-morbidity and its implications for drug and alcohol treatment. *Drug and Alcohol Dependence*, *49*, 61-69.

Kessler, R. C., Crum, R., Warner, C., Nelson, C., Schulenberg, J., & Anthony, J. C. (1997). Lifetime co-occurrence of DSM-III-R alcohol abuse and dependence with other psychiatric disorders in the National Comorbidity Survey. *Archives of General Psychiatry*, *54*, 313-321.

Kessler, R. C., McGonagle, K. A., Zhao, S., Nelson, C. B., Hughes, S., Eshleman, S., Wittchen, H., & Kendler, K. (1994). Lifetime and 12 month prevalence of DSM-III-R psychiatric disorders in the United States: Results from National Comorbidity Survey. *Archives of General Psychiatry*, *51*, 8-19.

Khantzian, E. J. (1990). Self-regulation and self-medication factors in alcoholism and the addictions: Similarities and differences. *Recent Developments in Alcoholism*, *8*, 255.

Kocsis, J. H., Markowitz, J. C., & Prien, R. F. (1990). Comorbidity of dysthymic disorder. In J. D. Maser & C. R. Cloninger (Eds.), *Comorbidity of mood and anxiety disorders* (pp. 317-328). Washington, DC: American Psychiatric Press.

Morse, J., & Field, P. (1995). *Qualitative research methods for health professionals.* Thousand Oaks, CA: Sage Publications.

Pokorny, A. D., Miller, B. A., & Kaplan, H. B. (1972). The brief MAST: A shortened version of the Michigan Alcoholism Screening Test. *American Journal of Psychiatry*, *129*, 342-345.

Schuckit, M. A., Tipp, M. E., Bulchoz, K. K., Nurnberger, J. I., Hesselbrock, C. M., Crowe, R. R., & Kramer, J. (1997). The lifetime rates of 3 major mood disorders and 4 major anxiety disorders in alcoholics and controls. *Addiction*, *92*, 1189-304.

Stewart, S. H., Brown, C. G., Theakston, J., Devoulyte, K., & Larsen, S. E. (2006). Why do women with alcohol problems binge eat? Exploring connections between binge eating and heavy drinking in women receiving treatment for alcohol problems. *Journal of Health Psychology*, *14*, 77-82.

Stewart, S. H., Conrod, P. J., Marlatt, G. A., Comeau, M. N., Thush, C., & Krank, M. (2005). New developments in prevention and early intervention for alcohol abuse in youth. *Alcoholism: Clinical and Experimental Research*, *29*, 278-286.

Stewart, S. H., & Israeli, A. L. (2003). Substance abuse and co-occurring psychiatric disorders in victims of intimate violence. In C. Wekerle & A. M. Wall (Eds.), *The violence and addiction equation: Theoretical and clinical issues in substance abuse and relationship violence* (pp. 98-122). New York: Brunner-Mazel.
Stoppard, J. M. (1999). Why new perspectives are needed for understanding depression in women. *Canadian Psychology, 40*, 79-90.
Strauss, A., & Corbin, J. (1990). *Basics of qualitative research: Grounded theory procedures and techniques*. Newbury Park, CA: Sage.
Weiss, R. D., Griffin, M. L., & Tobin, S. M. (1992). Drug abuse as self-medication for depression: An empirical study. *American Journal of Drug and Alcohol Abuse, 18*, 121-129.

Depressive Symptoms, Gender, and Sexual Risk Behavior Among African-American Adolescents: Implications for Prevention and Intervention

Keisha Carr Paxton, PhD

W. LaVome Robinson, PhD

INTRODUCTION

Recent statistics suggest that African-American adolescents are engaging in a number of behaviors that place them at high risk for unplanned/unwanted pregnancy and contracting sexually transmitted infections (STIs), including contracting the human immunodeficiency virus (HIV). African Americans comprise only 16% of the subpopulation of persons under the age of 18 years. (United States Census Bureau, 2003). However, African-American youths are disproportionately represented among cases of STIs, including HIV. The rates of chlamydia and gonorrhea for youths aged 15-19 have increased dramatically in recent years; however, the rates for African Americans in this age range far surpass those of their Caucasian and Latino peers (Centers for Disease Control and Prevention [CDC], 2004a). For example, the rate of chlamydia reported in 2003 for African-American youths 15-19 years of age was 1.5 and 3 times that of Caucasians and Latinos of the same age, respectively (CDC, 2004a). Compared to their Caucasian and Latino peers, African-American adolescents are more likely to have had sexual intercourse and to be currently sexually active (Blum et al., 2000; CDC, 2004b). African-American adolescents report earlier ages of sexual debut than their non-African-American counterparts (CDC, 2004b). Early involvement in sexual activity is associated with greater sexual risk behaviors (Black, Ricardo, & Stanton, 1997; Rodrigue, Tercyak, & Lescano, 1997); thus, African-American youths, relative to other youths, are at greater risk for related negative outcomes. Furthermore, African-American youths are more likely to report having had greater than four sexual partners during their lifetime, compared to Caucasian and Latino adolescents (CDC, 20004b). As the number of sexual partners increases, so does the risk of contracting an STI from an infected partner (Millstein, Moscicki, & Broering, 1993), rendering African-American adolescents as one of the most at-risk groups of youth.

From July, 2002 to June, 2003, African-American females with HIV mostly contracted the virus through heterosexual contact (CDC, 2004c); whereas, in the same year, African-American males with HIV contracted the virus mostly through homosexual contact (CDC, 2004c). These differences point to examination of sexual risk behaviors by gender, as gender suggests behavioral risk factor differences for African-American youths.

Another factor associated with risk for African-American youths is mental health. To date, there is relatively little research on the relationship between mental health and sexual activity among adolescents, particularly so for African-American adolescents. Most of the research examining mental health and sexual activity has been conducted on specialized adult samples (e.g., homosexual or bisexual Caucasian males) and has yielded mixed results. Dilley, McFarland, Sullivan, and Discepola (1998) examined psychosocial factors associated with unprotected anal intercourse in a primarily Caucasian sample of adult gay and bisexual males. They found no association between depressive symptomology and unprotected sexual activity. However, in a similar study, Perkins, Leserman, Murphy, and Evans (1993) found relationships between depressive symptomology, anger, and unprotected anal intercourse among gay males, such that high reports of anger and depressive symptomology were associated with high-risk sexual behavior. Although these studies were conducted on a very specific population and their results provide limited generalizability, the studies argue for the continued examination of the relationship between depressive symptomology and sexual risk behaviors.

Among adolescents, most of the research examining sexual behavior and depressive symptomology has been conducted on Caucasian samples. Whitbeck and colleagues (Whitbeck, Conger, & Kao, 1993; Whitbeck, Hoyt, Miller, & Kao, 1992; Whitbeck, Yoder, Hoyt, & Conger, 1999) produced several studies looking at the relationship between depressed affect, sexual behavior, and other variables among samples of Caucasian adolescents. In a longitudinal study, Whitbeck et al. (1993) found that parent-child interactions were negatively associated with depressed affect which, in turn, was positively associated with permissive sexual ideals and sexual behaviors. Another study by Whitbeck and colleagues (1992) found a significant negative relationship between the quality of parental relationship and depressive symptomology among both boys and girls sampled. However, depressive symptomology was related to sexual activity and alcohol use only in girls, suggesting that gender differences exist in how depressive symptomology relates to sexual activity among adolescents. Similarly, in a 1999 study, Whitbeck and colleagues also found gender differences in sexual activity and depressed affect, such that depressed affect increased the likelihood of early sexual behavior among females, but not males, again pointing to gender differences in this area.

In a relevant study of precursors to adolescent pregnancy among African-American females, researchers found that depressed affect in mid-adolescence was a risk factor for pregnancy between the ages of 15 and 19 (Miller-Johnson et al., 1999). While this study does not prove that depressed affect caused teen pregnancy among the girls surveyed, it does provide support for the possibility of a relationship between sexual risk behavior and depressive symptomology among African-American females.

The aforementioned studies support the relationship between sexual risk behavior and affective status among adolescents, particularly so for females. Given that depression is a common mental health concern during adolescence (Lewinsohn, Shankman, Gau, & Klein, 2004) and given the high rates of sexual activity among African-American adolescents, research in the area of depression and sexual activity among African-American youths is especially needed, as this relationship may be particularly informative to preventive intervention development. In light of the research, we hypothesized that within a sample of inner-city African-American adolescents: (1) males would report engaging in more sexual risk behavior than females, (2) higher levels of depressive symptomology would be significantly associated with higher levels of sexual risk behavior and depressive symptomology would be a stronger predictor of sexual risk behavior for females than for males.

METHOD

Participants

Participants were 1,970 inner-city African-American youths, in grades nine and eleven, from seven Midwestern public high schools. Over 90% of the student bodies of each school were African American. The age of the sample ranged from 13 to 18 years of age, with a mean age of 15.45 (*SD* = 1.17 years). Participants were recruited through a variety of means, including presentations in exclusively ninth grade and eleventh grade courses, presentations during assemblies, recruitment booths set up during nutrition and lunch breaks, and booths set up during report card pick up days and other school functions. Both student participation assent and parental consent were obtained. Participation rates as high as 75% were achieved in the targeted schools, which is impressive, given the high rate of absenteeism in these schools which are located in very turbulent neighborhoods. Of the seven schools, three had school-based health centers (SBHCs) and four did not. Although presence or absence of an SBHC was not the focus of this study, it deserves examination, as the exposure to such a resource may impact the findings of this study. SBHCs are health clinics located either on or near school premises providing a wide array of services from allied health professionals. These services range from conducting physicals to providing contraception and mental health services.

The sample was almost evenly split between males and females. Two-thirds of the sample was in the ninth grade and one-third was in the twelfth grade. Just over one-third (36.8%) attended a school with a school-based health center. Eighty percent of the sample endorsed at least one indicator of poverty. The majority of the sample (79.5%) reported being sexually active. Table 1 provides detailed descriptive information on the sample.

Measures

The current study was part of a larger study of adolescent health that consisted of 19 self-report measures. The measures presented are those that relate to the hypotheses for the current study. Demographic information was obtained via single-item questions assessing grade, gender (coded as males = 0 and females = 1), and race/ethnic background. Socioeconomic status was measured by endorsing at least one source of economic assistance (i.e., eligibility for free or reduced-price school lunch program, family receiving government assistance, unemployment as an income source, and receiving food stamps, coded as absent = 0 and present = 1). Schools also were coded to reflect presence or absence of SBHC (coded as no SBHC = 0 and SBHC = 1).

Center for Epidemiologic Studies–Depression Scale (CES-D). Depressive symptomology was assessed using the CES-D. The CES-D is a widely used 20-item scale assessing depressive symptomology. Each question

TABLE 1. Descriptive Information for the Sample (N = 1,970)

Category	%
Demographics	
Female	55.6
Male	44.4
9th grade	66.3
11th grade	33.3
School has SBHC	36.8
1 or more poverty indicators	80.2
Sexual Behavior	
Ever had sex	79.5
Sexually active before age 13	17.5
Four or more partners, lifetime	37.5
Depressive Symptomalogy	*Mean (SD)*
Females	19.5 (10.2)
Males	14.4 (8.00)
Total	17.3 (9.62)

Note. SBHC = school-based health center. SD = standard deviation.

asked participants to rate each symptom on a 4-point Likert scale, assessing how often during the past week they experienced each symptom. The questions strongly reflect diagnostic criteria for depression set by the American Psychiatric Association in the Diagnostic and Statistical Manual of Mental Disorders (3rd ed., rev., 1987). This measure has been shown to be valid for a variety of populations, including adolescents, in assessing depressive symptomology (Radloff, 1991). The CES-D has high internal consistency ranging from .85 to .90 and test-retest reliability ranging from .45 to .70 (Radloff, 1991). Internal consistency for the current sample was quite good ($\alpha = .81$).

Sexual behavior. Sexual risk behavior was assessed using 4 items taken from the Youth Risk Behavior Surveillance Survey (CDC, 1990, 1996, 1998), to form an index of sexual behavior. The domains of questions included whether or not participants had ever been sexually active, the age of sexual debut, the number of sexual partners in the past 3 months, and frequency of condom use. Responses were scored and summed to create a score of sexual risk, ranging from no risk (0) to highest risk (16). The item asking number of sexual partners during the last 3 months was used to assess the occurrence of recent sexual activity. Point values were assigned to each potential answer for the questions comprising the sexual risk behavior index. The test-retest reliability on these questions ranged from .59-.88 and the internal consistency for these items was .66 in the current sample.

Procedure

Surveys were administered in group sessions at the participants' respective schools. The surveys were divided into four sections and organized into four different versions to allow for counterbalancing of the instrument. The survey was read aloud by a member of the research team to control for differences in reading ability. Each participant completed the survey as it was read aloud.

Participants were given the complete instrument and asked to write their name on the initial page, which also had an identification number on it. They were then asked to remove that page and give it to the research staff. The survey also had the identification number on it and this number was used to match survey responses with archival data about participants.

Participants were told that their responses would be completely confidential and no school personnel would have access to the surveys. Survey administration took place in available classrooms that were free from distraction at each school. Completion of the survey took approximately one hour, so students were excused from two consecutive class periods to allow for the survey to be completed in one sitting. Upon completion of the survey, research staff collected the surveys and provided participants with non-monetary compensation (e.g., movie tickets). Prior to conduct, this study was approved by the Institutional Review Board at DePaul University.

RESULTS

The current study examined the link between sexual risk behavior and depressive symptoms among African-American inner-city adolescents in schools where some participants were exposed to school-based health centers (SBHCs) and other participants did not have SBHC services available at their school. As presence of an SBHC may confound results, this was controlled for in the analyses, as were grade and socioeconomic status.

Hypothesis I predicted that males would be more likely to engage in sexual-risk behaviors than females. To examine this hypothesis, a two-step multiple linear regression was conducted where sexual risk behavior was regressed on the control variables (e.g., grade, socioeconomic status, and presence of a school-based health center) and on gender. In the linear regression analysis, the control variables were entered on the first step and gender was entered on the second step. Gender significantly predicted sexual risk behavior above and beyond the effects of the control variables, with males more likely to engage in sexual risk behavior (Table 2). Furthermore, the inclusion of gender in the regression model accounted for significantly more variance (16.5%) in predicting sexual risk behavior than the control variables alone (0.5%).

Controlling for the effects of grade, socioeconomic status, and presence of a school-based health center, Hypothesis II stated that there would be a significant main effect for depressive symptomology predicting sexual risk behavior and that there would be a significant interaction for gender. To examine this hypothesis, a four-step multiple linear regression was conducted. The independent variables were entered in the following order: (a) control variables (e.g., grade, socioeconomic status,

TABLE 2. Multiple Linear Regression of Sexual Risk Behavior Regressed on Demographic Variables, Gender, Depressive Symptomology, and Gender by Depressive Symptomology Interaction (N = 1,843)

Variable	*Beta*	*SE*	β
Step 1			
Grade	–.35	.20	–.04
≥ 1 poverty indicators	–.33	.24	–.03
School has SBHC	.42	.20	.05*
R^2	.005		
Step 2			
Gender	–3.27	.17	–.40***
R^2	.165[a]		
Step 3			
Depressive symptomology	2.21E-02	.01	.05*
R^2	.168[a]		
Step 4			
Depressive symptomology x Gender	5.38E-02	.02	.17**
R^2	.171[a]		

Note. SBHC = school-based health center. *SE* = standard error. R^2 for each step is cumulative. [a] indicates significant increase in R^2 over previous block entered. *$p < .05$. **$p < .01$. ***$p < .001$.

and presence of school-based health center), (b) gender, (c) depressive symptomology, and (d) interaction of gender and depressive symptomology. The purpose of entering the independent variables in this order was to determine the impact of depressive symptomology above and beyond any impact of the control variables and gender and to determine the effect of an interaction for gender and depressive symptomology above and beyond that of the two independently and of the control variables.

Gender, depressive symptomology, and the interaction of gender and depressive symptomology were found to be significant predictors of sexual risk behavior (Table 2). Males were more likely to engage in greater sexual risk behavior than females. In addition, participants endorsing a greater amount of depressive symptomology were more likely to be involved in sexual risk behaviors. Moreover, the interaction suggests that depressive symptomology was a stronger predictor of sexual risk behavior for females than for males. There were significant increases in R^2 between steps 1 ($R^2 = .005$) and 2 ($R^2 = .165$), steps 2 ($R^2 = .165$) and 3 ($R^2 = .168$), and steps 3 ($R^2 = .168$) and 4 (final $R^2 = .171$), suggesting that the inclusion of depressive symptomology provided a better model of predicting sexual risk above that of gender and that the gender by depressive symptomology interaction term provided a better model for the prediction of sexual risk behavior than gender and depressive symptomology alone.

In supplemental analyses, we ran two separate regressions for males and females to confirm that gender was a moderating variable. The regression of sexual risk behavior on depression for the female group was significant and the same regression analysis for the male group was insignificant, thus confirming that depressive symptomology was indeed a significant predictor of sexual risk behavior among females.

DISCUSSION

This study sought to add to the current literature base on adolescent sexuality by examining the relationship between depressive symptomology and sexual risk behavior. This study is among the first to show a relationship between depressive symptomology and sexual risk behavior within a sample of African-American adolescents. The findings of this study have important implications for intervention development and future research.

Most importantly, this study found a significant relationship between depressive symptomology and sexual activity. Consistent with research on sexual activity and depressive symptomology among Caucasian youths (e.g., Whitbeck et al., 1992), gender differences were found in the current study, such that as depressive symptomology increases among females, there is greater sexual risk behavior. However, in the current study this relationship did not exist for males. The research on depressive symptomology and gender generally supports that females have a higher prevalence of depressive symptomology than males (Nolen-Hoeksema, 1994; Nolen-Hoeksema & Girgus, 1994) and the present study supports that depressive symptomology is linked to sexual risk behavior among African-American adolescent females. Thus, efforts to reduce sexual risk behavior among African-American females should consider the reduction of mental health concomitants such as depressive symptomology, in addition to the more traditional approaches to sexual risk reduction.

Although a causal direction cannot be inferred, as the data is correlational, the link between depressive symptomology and sexual risk behavior among African-American adolescent females is nonetheless notable. The findings strongly point to the inclusion of a mental health component in adolescent sexual risk reduction programs, particularly so for African-American adolescent females. Conversely, in group-based and individual therapy with depressed African-American adolescent females, it may be necessary to address involvement in a variety of risk behaviors, particularly sexual risk behavior. The current findings, as well as previous research, point to the need for future research addressing the temporal relationship between depressive symptomology and sexual risk behavior, especially among African-American adolescent females.

The unique social ecology of African-American youths may be central to understanding the apparent gender differences in their sexual risk behavior and the design of prevention programs. The majority of the present sample came from urban neighborhoods with a fair amount of gang activity and community violence. Research supports the relationship between exposure to violence and depressive symptomology among African-American females (e.g., Moses, 1999). It may well be that depressive symptomology mediates a relationship between exposure to violence and sexual risk behavior among African-American adolescent females. This is an area for future research that would ultimately inform prevention intervention development.

Similarly, a qualitative study of African-American adolescents found that many of the females surveyed stated that either they or their female peers engaged in sexual activity as a means of survival (Vera, Reese, Paikoff, & Jarrett, 1996). That is, in some neighborhoods with a great deal of violence (e.g., thefts, muggings, homicides, weapon usage, fighting, and gang activity), girls may feel it necessary to engage in sexual intercourse with male gang members in exchange for protection. The effects of exposure to violence may also manifest as depressive symptomology. As such, protecting herself from sexually transmitted diseases or unwanted pregnancy may be the least of the girls' concerns. This study further argues the importance of including exposure to violence, depressive symptomology, and sexual risk behavior link in the design of prevention interventions.

As with any research there were limitations in the conduct of the current study that should be noted. Measurement of various constructs is an important area to consider in this study. Foremost, sexual risk behavior is difficult to quantify. Of the existing research in this area, there is no widely used standard measure of sexual risk behavior for youth. Consequently, researchers often utilize one or two items to assess this behavior (e.g., Fisher & Feldman, 1998; Upchurch, Aneshensel, Sucoff, & Storms, 1999) or they utilize self-developed scales lacking rigorous examination of their psychometric properties (e.g., Fergusson & Lynskey, 1996; Stanton et al., 1993). This study utilized items from the Youth Risk Behavior Surveillance Survey (CDC, 1990, 1996, 1998) that are widely used on diverse samples of adolescents; however, an alternative, standardized measure of sexual risk may have yielded other results.

The current study obtained data via self-report measures. Limitations of self-report data include subjective interpretation, possible low correlation with concurrent behavioral measures, and potential bias toward social desirability (Nietzel, Bernstein, & Russell, 1988). To reduce faking and social desirability, a number of questions assessing consistency of responding were embedded within the larger survey (but not in the measures used in these analyses); nonetheless the potential of faking or socially desirable responding cannot be eliminated with absolute certainty. In addition to the above limitations, depressive symptomology and sexual behaviors were assessed for different time periods, which may impact results. Specifically, depressive symptomology was assessed for the week prior to the study and sexual behavior was assessed over the participant's lifetime. Finally, the fact that only youths attending school participated in the study limits the generalizability of the findings.

Overall, however, the findings of the present study are informative and augment the current research base pertaining to the relationship between depressive symptomology and sexual risk behavior among African-American adolescent females. Despite the aforementioned study limitations, the implications of the current study for prevention intervention development and future research are notable. This study is an important step toward the identification of emotional factors associated with risky sexual behavior among African-American adolescent females, a population of youth at high risk (Barber, Hall & Armistead, 2003; DiClemente et al., 2004) and in great need.

REFERENCES

American Psychiatric Association. (1987). *Diagnostic and statistical manual of mental disorders* (3rd ed., rev.). Washington, DC: Author.

Barber, C., Hall, J., & Armistead, L. (2003). Parent-adolescent relationship and adolescent psychological functioning among African-American female adolescents: Self-esteem as a mediator. *Journal of Child and Family Studies, 12*, 361-374.

Black, M. M., Ricardo, I. B., & Stanton, B. (1997). Social and psychological factors associated with AIDS risk behaviors among low-income, urban, African-American adolescents. *Journal of Research on Adolescence, 7*, 173-195.

Blum, R. W., Deuhring, T., Shew, M. L., Bearinger, L. H., Sieving, R. E., & Resnick, M. D. (2000). The effects of race/ethnicity, income, and family structure on adolescent risk behaviors. *American Journal of Public Health, 90*, 1879-1884.

Centers for Disease Control and Prevention. (1990). *Development of the youth risk behavior survey questionnaire.* Atlanta: Author.

Centers for Disease Control and Prevention. (1996). Youth risk behavior surveillance–United States, 1995. *Morbidity and Mortality Weekly Report. CDC Surveillance Summaries, 47*, 1-84.

Centers for Disease Control and Prevention. (1998). Youth risk behavior surveillance–United States, 1997. *Morbidity and Mortality Weekly Report. CDC Surveillance Summaries, 47*, 1-89.

Centers for Disease Control and Prevention. (2004a, September). *Sexually transmitted disease surveillance, 2003.* Atlanta, GA: U.S. Department of Health and Human Services.

Centers for Disease Control and Prevention. (2004b). Youth risk behavior surveillance–United States, 2003. *Morbidity and Mortality Weekly Report. CDC Surveillance Summaries, 53*(SS-2), 1-100.

Centers for Disease Control and Prevention (2004c). *U.S. HIV and AIDS surveillance report, 2003.* Atlanta: U.S. Department of Health and Human Services.

DiClemente, R. J., Wingood, G. M., Harrington, K. F., Lang, D. L., Davies, S. L., Hook, E. W. et al. (2004). Efficacy of an HIV prevention intervention for African-American adolescent girls: A randomized controlled trial. *Journal of the American Medical Association, 292*, 171-179.

Dilley, J. W., McFarland, W., Sullivan, P., & Discepola, M. (1998). Psychosocial correlates of unprotected anal sex in a cohort of gay men attending an HIV-negative support group. *AIDS Education and Prevention, 10*, 317-326.

Fergusson, D. M., & Lynskey, M. T. (1996). Alcohol misuse and adolescent sexual behaviors and risk-taking. *Pediatrics, 98*, 91-96.

Fisher, L., & Feldman, S. S. (1998). Familial antecedents of young adult health risk behavior: A longitudinal study. *Journal of Family Psychology, 12*, 66-80.

Lewinsohn, P. M., Shankman, S. A., Gau, J. M., & Klein, D. N. (2004). The prevalence and co-morbidity of subthreshold psychiatric conditions. *Psychological Medicine, 34*, 613-622.

Miller-Johnson, S., Winn, D. M., Coie, J., Maumary-Gremaud, A., Hyman, C., Robert, T., & Lochman, J. (1999). Motherhood during the teen years: A developmental perspective on risk factors for childbearing. *Development and Psychopathology, 11*, 85-100.

Millstein, S. G., Moscicki, A. B., & Broering, J. M. (1993). Female adolescents at high, moderate, and low risk for exposure to HIV: Differences in knowledge, beliefs, and behaviors. *Journal of Adolescent Health, 15*, 133-142.

Moses, A. (1999). Exposure to violence, depression, and hostility in a sample of inner city high school youth. *Journal of Adolescence, 22*, 21-32.

Nietzel, M. T., Bernstein, D. A., & Russell, R. L. (1988). Assessment of anxiety and fear. In A. S. Bellack & M. Hersen (Eds.), *Behavioral assessment: A practical handbook* (3rd ed., pp. 280-312). NY: Pergamon Press.

Nolen-Hoeksema, S. (1994). An interactive model for the emergence of gender differences in depression in adolescence. *Journal of Research on Adolescence, 4*, 519-534.

Nolen-Hoeksema, S., & Girgus, J. S. (1994). The emergence of gender differences in depression during adolescence. *Psychological Bulletin, 115*, 424-443.

Perkins, D. O., Leserman, J., Murphy, C., & Evans, D. L. (1993). Psychosocial predictors of high-risk sexual behavior among HIV-negative homosexual men. *AIDS Education and Prevention, 5*, 141-152.

Radloff, L. S. (1991). The use of the Center for Epidemiologic Studies Depression Scale in adolescents and young adults. *Journal of Youth and Adolescents, 20*, 149-166.

Rodrigue, J. R., Tercyak, K. P., & Lescano, C. M. (1997). Health promotion in minority adolescents: Emphasis on sexually transmitted diseases and the human immunodeficiency virus. In D. K. Wilson, J. R. Rodrigue, & W. C. Taylor (Eds.), *Health-promoting and health-compromising behaviors among minority adolescents* (pp. 87-105). Washington, DC: American Psychological Association.

Stanton, B. F., Black, M., Feigelman, S., Kaljee, L., Keane, V., & Nesbitt, R. (1995). Development of a culturally, theoretically and developmentally based survey instrument for assessing of risk behaviors among African Americans living in urban low- income neighborhoods. *AIDS Education and Prevention, 7*, 160-177.

United States Census Bureau, Current Population Survey (2003, March). Racial Statistics Branch, Population Division. Retrieved December 10, 2004 from: http://www.census.gov/population/socdemo/race/black/ppl-164/tab01.pdf.

Upchurch, D.M., Aneshensel, C.S., Sucoff, C.A., & Storms, L.L. (1999). Neighborhood and family contexts of adolescent sexual activity. *Journal of Marriage and the Family, 61*, 920-933.

Vera, E. M., Reese, L. E., Paikoff, R. L., & Jarrett, R. L. (1996). Contextual factors of sexual risk-taking in urban African-American preadolescent children, In B. J. R. Leadbeater & N. Way (Eds.), *Urban girls: Resisting stereotypes, creating identities* (pp. 291-304). New York: New York University Press.

Whitbeck, L. B., Conger, R. D., & Kao, M. (1993). The influence of parental support, depressed affect, and peers on the sexual behaviors of adolescents girls. *Journal of Family Issues*, *14*, 261-278.

Whitbeck, L. B., Hoyt, D. R., Miller, M., & Kao, M. (1992). Parental support, depressed affect, and sexual experiences among adolescents. *Youth and Society*, *24*, 166-177.

Whitbeck, L. B., Yoder, K. A., Hoyt, D. R., & Conger, R. D. (1999). Early adolescent sexual activity: A developmental study. *Journal of Marriage and the Family*, *61*, 934-946.

The Needs of Depressed Women: Perspectives of Family Physicians

Janet M. Stoppard, PhD

Roanne Thomas-MacLean, PhD

Baukje Miedema, PhD
Sue Tatemichi, MD, CCFP, FCFP

INTRODUCTION

It is estimated by the World Health Organization that depression accounts for approximately 25% of all visits by people to health care professionals (Gerrity, Cole, Deitrich, & Barrett, 1999), and family physicians are most often the initial health care contact for depressed patients (Williams et al., 1999). Given their role in delivery of primary health care, family physicians represent a special opportunity to address intervention and prevention issues in the community with respect to depression (Docherty, 1997). Despite the fact that most primary care physicians report treating depressed patients in their offices, very few studies have addressed the issue directly from the standpoint of family physicians.

To address this gap in knowledge, we conducted a study with family physicians in a province in Atlantic Canada about their experiences in providing care to depressed patients. Given that epidemiological studies indicate higher rates of depression among women than men in community samples (Health Canada, 2002; Stewart, Gucciardi, & Grace, 2004), women are likely to predominate among the depressed patients seen by family physicians. Although fewer than half of individuals in Canada who meet diagnostic criteria for depression receive treatment, women are more likely than men to receive treatment and to be treated by a family physician (Diverty & Beaudet, 1997).

A recent survey of family physicians in the UK indicated that medication was the treatment most often used with depressed patients (Telford, Hutchinson, Jones, Rix, & Howe, 2002). In Canada, antidepressants are also the primary mode of treatment for individuals diagnosed with a depressive disorder who seek care from a health professional (Patten & Beck, 2004). Less is known, however, about use of other treatment approaches, such as counselling or psychological therapy, in the primary care setting. At the same time, physicians identify lack of ready access to these forms of intervention as a barrier to provision of care for depressed patients (Miedema, Tatemichi, Thomas-MacLean, & Stoppard, 2004; Telford et al., 2002). Exploration of the experiences of family physicians in providing care to depressed women would contribute to knowledge about physicians' decision-making in relation to interventions with depressed patients. More specifically, the perspective of family physicians provides a unique vantage point from which to investigate the needs of depressed women, both in the primary care setting and in the wider community.

METHOD

Study Setting

The hospital region in which the study took place has a catchment population of approximately 170,000, with about half of this population being characterized as rural. Approximately 100 family physicians practise within this hospital region. Almost all have private offices and are reimbursed on a fee-for-service basis by the provincial government.

Recruitment and Selection of Participants

All family physicians practising in the hospital region were invited to participate in the study. From the 40 physicians who responded, 20 were selected for interview using a purposive sampling technique to ensure diversity of perspectives. The criteria used to select interview participants were: gender, location of practice (urban/rural), and year of graduation from medical school. Physicians were offered an honorarium to reimburse their time and overhead costs. The final interview sample consisted of 9 men and 11 women. Eleven physicians practised in urban areas (4 male and 7 female) and 9 in rural areas (5 male and 4 female). Eight of the participants graduated from medical school prior to 1980 (7 male and 1 female), five in the 1980s (1 male and 4 female), and seven completed their education in the 1990s (1 male and 6 female). All of the physicians indicated that they were actively involved with diagnosis and treatment of depressed patients.

Procedures

The interviews were conducted by one team member (RTM), who piloted the interview guide with another team member (ST). Interviews lasted approximately one hour and were conducted in person. All but two of the interviews were conducted in physicians' offices. The interviews followed a semi-structured format, using both formal (i.e., previously constructed) and informal (e.g., asking for specific examples) probes. Interview questions addressed the following topics: demographic information and practice characteristics, prevalence of depression in the physician's practice, diagnostic procedures with depressive conditions, treatment of depressed patients, and systemic issues in provision of care to depressed patients. Although the term "depression" was used by the interviewer, a formal definition was not provided. Saturation (i.e., the repetition of key ideas) was reached within 15 interviews. Five additional interviews were conducted to ensure sample diversity. Each interview was audiotaped and transcribed verbatim.

The first stage of the analysis involved use of NVivo software (QSR International, 2000) to retrieve transcript segments in which a physician discussed depressed women or girls directly or where female gender was clearly implied. This material was then analyzed thematically with respect to physicians' views on the causes of women's depression and their treatment strategies with depressed women. One team member (JMS) generated analytic themes and the other team members reviewed the themes and provided input on coherence, or validity, of the analysis (Willig, 2001). Analytic categories were generated through attention to recurrent thematic content both within and across transcripts, an approach to qualitative analysis that has been widely used in social science research (Willig, 2001).

RESULTS

Female physicians were more likely than male physicians to discuss depressed women during the interviews. Although both male and female physicians had treated depressed women, female physicians were more likely to report that they saw primarily women in their practice. In preliminary coding of the transcripts, text segments were coded into one of three "nodes," labelled Female, Male and Neutral. When the physicians referred to patient gender, female patients were mentioned specifically or female gender implied much more often than male patients or male gender were.[1]

Two main themes emerged from the analysis. One focused on physicians' understanding of the causes of women's depression and the other was concerned with treatment strategies used by physicians with depressed women. The first theme addressed physicians' views on the reasons that women seen in their practice had become depressed, rather than their knowledge of formal theories of depression. Thus, we were interested in how physicians' understanding of women's depression was shaped by their experience in the context of providing care to women patients. Similarly, the theme concerning physicians' treatment strategies with depressed women addressed treatment approaches they reported using, rather than actual usage rates of specific treatments with depressed patients.

Physicians' Views on the Causes of Women's Depression: Stress Arising From Social Factors

When discussing depressed women patients, physicians frequently mentioned sources of stress arising from social influences in women's lives as precipitants of depression. Within this overarching theme, three sub-themes were identified: social influences in the context of women's roles in the family; social influences specific to their lives as women; and, social factors that limited women's access to practical resources for addressing sources of stress in their lives.

Family-related stress. Physicians identified responsibilities related to providing care to family members as a source of stress for women, particularly when such care giving was combined with paid employment.

> The multi-tasking, the perceived need to be something for everybody, to not only be a good mother but also to bring in some income and also be the person who keeps the house tidy and keeps the kids organized for school . . . I think there are a lot of pressures that women feel. (FU1)[2]

The challenges faced by women raising children on their own were identified by physicians as being particularly stressful.

> . . . so if you have some lady who is raising a couple of kids . . . and she's working in a store or as a waitress, she doesn't have time or support to deal with a kid . . . that person, they need help. (MU1)

Gender-specific stress. Physicians identified low income as a source of stress specific to women, especially for those raising children on their own. A woman's financial dependence on her spouse, including the spouse's control of her access to money, was another gender-specific stressor identified by physicians.

> I had a patient come in last week and she works for I think six dollars per hour and her husband makes seventy to eighty thousand a year and yet forces her to put her money into the family pot and she doesn't feel as though she can even have a coffee without going to him and asking for five dollars . . . and over the years that erodes self-esteem to the point that she feels that she is nothing . . . (FU1)

Other gender-specific sources of stress were abuse by a partner (including control of a woman's access to money) and body-image concerns related to weight and appearance. Body-image concerns were often mentioned in the context of treatment decisions when weight gain was a factor in deciding which antidepressant to prescribe.

> Often times the people I'm seeing, females, are at least a little bit overweight and there are some self-esteem issues generally arising from that so when you tell them they're going to possibly gain weight with the tricyclics they're not all that happy to think about that so they usually say, no thank you. (FU1)

Practical sources of stress. Physicians also identified practical barriers women faced in engaging in activities that could help to reduce the stressfulness of their everyday lives. These were barriers created by lack of access to resources such as transportation or child care, which would allow women to make use of community services, including recreational and other self-care activities (e.g., mental health services). These practical sources of stress were usually linked by physicians to family-related or gender-specific sources of stress.

> . . . if you don't have a car . . . if your husband is being abusive . . . and doesn't allow you access or . . . wants to control every activity that you do, then you're not going to get to (nearby town). I mean it may as well be Vancouver. (FU6)

Physicians' Treatment Strategies with Depressed Women[3]

In line with their perceptions of stress as a precipitant of women's depression, the physicians identified various support services in the community that, if available, would help to reduce stress for depressed women. Child-care services, for instance, would enable women caring for children at home to have some time to engage in recreational activities and to socialize with friends. Self-help groups, where women could meet with others living in similar situations, were also seen as likely to be helpful.

> . . . to open up at a discussion group where 20 women could all be voicing the same thing, yeah . . . she simply needed validation that what she is feeling is normal . . . . that would be a great thing if they could do that in some kind of a group or forum so that they don't have to find out from us. (FU1)

Physicians' intervention strategies with women patients fell into two main categories: alleviating depressive symptoms and feelings of distress and reducing sources of stress in women's lives.

Alleviating depressive symptoms and distress. The treatment strategy mentioned most often by the physicians was use of antidepressants. Medication was seen as the first-line of treatment, either alone or in conjunction with referral for counselling or psychological therapy. One purpose of prescribing an antidepressant was to increase a woman's energy and mood levels before seeing a counsellor.

> If you're feeling the way that they are sometimes when they come for the first appointment, I mean they don't want to cook supper . . . . So in that situation I'll say let's get started today on medication and you make the appointment [with a psychologist] knowing that you won't see somebody probably for 2-3 weeks because by the time you are feeling better or starting to see some improvement, you'll have the physical and mental energy to attack some of those issues. (FU6)

If a physician decided that a woman would benefit from counselling or psychological therapy, she was usually referred to a service in the local community (either a mental health centre or a counsellor or psychologist in private practice), rather than providing this form of treatment themselves.

> If I try to do counselling with them and it doesn't work, okay, then they can't come back to me with those same complaints because my answer then is going to be "Well, have you done your homework, have you thought about this, what can you do to change it?" It changes the relationship between me and them. Now if I send them to a psychologist and things are not going well, then they can just leave the psychologist, they can just break off that relationship. It's not the same as breaking it off with your family doctor. Now suddenly they have to change practices, they have to find a new doctor because they can't admit that they're not willing to do this. (FR1)

When prescribing an antidepressant drug, the physician's choice was often shaped by a woman's concerns about side effects, such as weight gain or loss of sexual interest, especially with younger women.

> . . . the side-effects profile is certainly a biggie . . . if it's a young girl and the first thing she says is I don't want to gain weight, okay, and then I'm going to stay away from a couple of medications that I feel . . . at least in my experience, cause weight gain. (FU4)

A physician's choice of which antidepressant to prescribe was also influenced by a patient's ability to pay for drugs. Cost-related and structural issues in the delivery of primary care services were identified by the physicians that placed limits on the treatment strategies available to them. Although not specific to women patients, finding ways to overcome such barriers (e.g., by accessing pharmaceutical companies' compassionate care programs) added to the workloads of already busy physicians (cf. Miedema et al., 2004).

Stress reduction strategies. Physicians attempted to reduce sources of stress in women patients' lives by addressing the sources directly or by advising patients on lifestyle changes with the aim of reducing stress in their lives. As one physician said:

> I want to reduce the stresses that are aggravating this . . . a spouse assaulting them in some way, so you kind of reduce those things. (MU1)

Another physician gave the following examples of the kind of lifestyle changes she recommended to patients:

> The most recent case I can think of is a young woman with multiple stressors, many children, relationship issues, previous history of depression and so on and had also taken on a very major educational challenge in writing her thesis and just maybe suggesting to her that she put that on hold for awhile. . . . I find it's typically that type of thing–lightening the load a little bit, what can you do differently to what can you get those around you to do differently . . . (FU3)

DISCUSSION

Although the interviews with physicians did not focus specifically on women, women patients were mentioned frequently in the examples the physicians gave, particularly in the interviews with female physicians. In the initial coding of transcripts for gender-related content, we found that female patients were mentioned explicitly, or female gender was implied, more often than was the case for male or gender-neutral patient references. One explanation for this finding is that the interview sample consisted of slightly more female physicians (11) than male physicians (9) and the female physicians were more likely to report that they saw primarily women in their practice. At the same time, the more frequent mention of female patients by these physicians is in keeping with epidemiological findings indicating higher rates of depression among women than men in community samples (Stewart et al., 2004).

A recurrent theme in the physicians' accounts was the role of stress in women's lives as a precipitant of depression. Women's depression was attributed to stress arising from social factors in the context of their lives *as women*. Sources of stress identified by the physicians were related either to women's family roles or were gender-specific, and also arose from practical barriers which set limits on women's ability to engage in activities to reduce stress in their everyday lives. To some degree, these social sources of stress were interlinked, so that a woman might be restricted in her ability to engage in activities that would improve her well-being (e.g., exercising at the gym) because she lacked access to child care services and transportation, which in turn were due to her low income. For married women, such stressors could be exacerbated by having an abusive spouse who was controlling of a woman's access to such resources as transportation and money. The lives of women raising children on their own were identified by physicians as being particularly stressful, because of a woman's need to work outside the home to support herself and her children.

In line with these perceptions, physicians' treatment strategies with depressed women had a dual focus on alleviating depressive symptoms and distress and addressing sources of stress. Antidepressant medication was usually the first line of treatment for depressive symptoms. If a physician planned to refer a woman for counselling or psychotherapy, an antidepressant might be prescribed in order to increase her energy and mood levels before seeing a mental health practitioner in the community. Physicians also attempted to reduce stress in the lives of women patients by providing support to those coping with an abusive partner or recommending lifestyle changes with the aim of making their lives less stressful.

Physicians' attempts to reduce stress were restricted to addressing fairly immediate sources of stress, such as an abusive spouse, or providing advice on how a woman could "lighten" her load by cutting back on activities or enlisting the help of other family members. Such strategies are similar to findings by Stoppard and Gammell (2003) in an interview study with women about their experience of being treated for depression. Stoppard and Gammell found that women were often encouraged by their doctors to reduce their involvement in activities outside the home. For instance, a woman with a full-time job might switch to part-time employment. Although only one physician interviewed in the present study mentioned recommending to a woman patient that she cut back on her activities outside the home (by postponing an educational endeavour), the physicians' comments seemed to imply that stress in women patients' lives arose from trying to do too much. In their efforts to lighten a woman's load, physicians may unintentionally convey the idea that women should cut back on activities outside the home, a strategy in keeping with the selfless and nurturing "good woman" ideal that depressed women are likely to endorse (Lafrance, 2003). At the same time, the physicians also recognized a need for improved social resources within the community, such as child care services and support groups that would not only benefit depressed women, but would reduce stress in women's lives more generally.

Implications for Delivery of Primary Health Care Services

The physicians identified structural and other barriers (e.g., cost of medication) that affected their ability to treat depressed patients. Although these barriers were not specific to women patients, their impact is likely to be heightened for women because they involve the same factors that may bring depressed women to a physician's office in the first place. Thus, a woman's lack of access to social resources such as child care services, transportation and money may create stress in her life and also prevent her from receiving treatment for depression.

Although the physicians who participated in this study drew on a variety of treatment strategies with depressed patients, both male and female physicians relied primarily on antidepressant drugs. Such strategies included prescription of an antidepressant combined with supportive counselling and advice on lifestyle changes, usually with the aim of reducing family-related sources of stress in a woman's life. None of the physicians used psychological interventions, such as cognitive therapy, in their own practice, although one physician reported that she had attempted to do so earlier in her career. When a physician determined that a depressed patient would benefit from counselling or psychological therapy, referral was made to a service in the community. At the same time, physicians also identified problems in accessing services in the community, because of long waiting lists or cost (cf. Miedema et al., 2004). Thus, while the physicians recognized the potential usefulness of non-medical forms of intervention, their ability to incorporate these approaches into the treatment of depressed women was hampered by lack of resources, both on the part of patients (inability to pay for private services) and in the community (lack of publicly-funded services). This situation adds to the complexity of treating depression in the primary care setting, because the structural limitations of medicine are combined with the social factors associated with gender inequality.

One strategy not mentioned by these physicians was in-house provision of counselling or psychological services, an approach reported by family physicians in the UK (Telford et al., 2002). A shift to incorporate such arrangements in the setting in which the present study took place would require structural changes in the funding and delivery of primary health care.[4] Nonetheless, recognition by physicians of the role of social factors in women's depression points to a need to broaden current approaches to treatment of depression in the primary care setting by making greater use of psychosocial forms of intervention.

The term "counselling" was used by physicians in a fairly generic way to refer to any intervention involving a helping relationship between a patient and a mental health professional. Such nonspecific use of the term counselling may reflect service availability in the local community, rather than lack of knowledge by physicians about psychological approaches to intervention. However, these physicians seemed largely unaware of the proven effectiveness of cognitive therapy in the treatment of depression, both alone or when combined with antidepressant medication (DeRubeis et al., 2005).

Implications for Community-Based Services

In keeping with their views on the social causes of women's depression, physicians identified resources in the community, such as child care services and support groups, which would be helpful in reducing stress in the lives of depressed women. More generally, the physicians' observations underscore the need for improved services in support of care giving activities within the family. Women continue to be the major providers of care to family members and, increasingly, to an extended family that encompasses elderly relatives. For women caring for young children at home, such support needs could be met through increased availability of child care services, either through formal service provision or more informal arrangements. One physician identified a need for child sitting services and suggested a cooperative approach where women could share in such services as required.

The physicians also identified a need for improved public transportation to enable women to access mental health services and to participate in recreational activities. Such services are particularly crucial for women living in rural areas because health and leisure services are more likely to be located in urban centres. At the same time, service providers should be encouraged to pursue outreach activities to meet the needs of those living in rural areas. Lack of access to counselling services, in particular, was identified by the physicians as a serious concern. Support groups, where women caring for young children at home could meet others in the same situation, would help to address the social isolation that can foster feelings of depression.

CONCLUSION

Despite an emphasis on biomedical approaches to depression in their training, the physicians in this study recognized both psychological and social aspects of women's depression. Yet, health care services in the region where these physicians practise do not support the type of interventions that physicians identified as being needed. Moreover, physicians' ability to provide treatment to depressed women is circumscribed by structural factors within society that shape women's lives and which lie largely beyond the scope of family physicians to influence or change. Family physicians hold a unique position in their capacity to intervene in social processes likely to engender stress in the lives of women patients, a position that could be strengthened by broadening current approaches to depression to include psychosocial perspectives in addition to medical forms of intervention. Physicians' identification of sources of stress in women's lives as being linked to their becoming depressed points to a move in this direction within the primary care setting. More generally, our findings support efforts to develop multidisciplinary approaches to delivery of primary health care in conjunction with community-based interventions for addressing women's depression.

NOTES

1. Only one male physician, who practised in a rural area and graduated from medical school before 1980, did not mention female patients during the interview.
2. Physicians are designated in the following way: F or M indicates physician gender and R or U indicates rural or urban location of practice. Physicians were numbered consecutively within each gender/location group. Thus, FU1 denotes the first female physician with an urban practice.
3. Although all of the physicians discussed their treatment approaches with depressed patients during the interview, female physicians were more likely to give examples of treating women patients, whereas male physicians were less likely to specify patient gender in their treatment examples. This pattern is reflected in the predominance of excerpts from interviews with female physicians selected to illustrate analytic themes.
4. In Canada, the funding and delivery of primary health care is primarily a provincial responsibility.

REFERENCES

DeRubeis, R. J., Hollon, S. D., Amsterdam, J. D., Shelton, R. C., Young, P. R., Salomon, R. M. et al. (2005). Cognitive therapy versus medications in the treatment of moderate to severe depression. *Archives of General Psychiatry*, *62*, 409-416.

Diverty, B., & Beaudet, M. P. (1997). Depression: An undertreated disorder? *Health Reports*, *8*, 9-18.

Docherty, J. P. (1997). Barriers to the diagnosis of depression in primary care. *Journal of Clinical Psychiatry*, *58*(Suppl. 1), 5-10.

Gerrity, M. S., Cole, S. A., Dietrich, A. J., & Barrett, J. E. (1999). Improving the recognition and management of depression: Is there a role for physician education? *Journal of Family Practice*, *48*, 949-957.

Health Canada. (2002). *A report on mental illnesses in Canada.* Ottawa: Author.

Lafrance, M. N. (2003). *Struggling for legitimacy: Women's experiences of recovery from depression.* Unpublished doctoral dissertation, University of New Brunswick.

Miedema, B., Tatemichi, S., Thomas-MacLean, R., & Stoppard, J. M. (2004). Barriers to treating depression in the family physician's office. *Canadian Journal of Community Mental Health*, *23*, 37-46.

Patten, S. B., & Beck, C. A. (2004). Major depression and mental health care utilization in Canada: 1994 to 2000. *Canadian Journal of Psychiatry*, *49*, 303-309.
QSR International. (2000). *NVivo qualitative data analysis program version 1.3.* Melbourne, Australia: Author.
Stewart, D. E., Gucciardi, E., & Grace, S. L. (2004). Depression. *BMC Women's Health*, *4*(Suppl. 1):S19. Retrieved February 26, 2005, from http://www.biomedcentral.com/1472-6874/4/S1/S19.
Stoppard, J. M., & Gammell, D. J. (2003). Depressed women's treatment experiences: Exploring themes of medicalization and empowerment. In J. M. Stoppard & L. M. McMullen (Eds.), *Situating sadness: Women and depression in social context* (pp. 39-61). New York: New York University Press.
Telford, R., Hutchinson, A., Jones, R., Rix, S., & Howe, A. (2002). Obstacles to effective treatment of depression: A general practice perspective. *Family Practice*, *19*, 45-52.
Williams, J. W., Mulrow, C. D., Kroenke, K., Dhanda, R., Badgett, R. G., Omori, D. et al. (1999). Case-finding for depression in primary care: A randomized trial. *American Journal of Medicine*, *106*, 36-43.
Willig, C. (2001). *Introducing qualitative research in psychology: Adventures in theory and method.* Buckingham, UK: Open University Press.

Community Service Providers' Conceptualizations of the Needs and Services of Depressed Rural Women

Mandy York, MSc

Peter Horvath, PhD

Mandy York, MSc, is Doctoral Candidate, Counselling Psychology Doctorate Pro gram, Department of Educational Psychology, University of Alberta, 6-102 Education North, Edmonton, AB, Canada T6G 2G5 (E-mail: myork@ualberta.ca).

Address correspondence to: Peter Horvath, PhD, Professor, Department of Psychology, Acadia University, Wolfville, NS, Canada B4P 2R6 (Email: Peter.Horvath@ acadiau.ca).

The authors gratefully acknowledge the support of a Community Research Alliance Grant from the Nova Scotia Health Research Foundation in the development of the measures used in this study. Pans of this study were based on the master's thesis of the first author.

INTRODUCTION

Two major barriers have been discussed in the literature as standing in the way of better services for depressed women in rural communities. One issue has to do with obstacles to accessing services and treatment (Fox, Blank, Rovnyak, & Barnett, 2001; Logan, Stevenson, Evans, & Leukefeld, 2004). The other issue has to do with the availability of appropriate and effective services for depressed women (Graveline, 1990; Hughes & McCormack, 2000; Raingruber, 2002). Community groups and agencies are in a position to extend their services to depressed women in the community and to help remove these barriers. However, their involvement depends to a considerable extent on their cooperation. Community service providers' conceptualizations of mental-disorders and their treatment are important because they could influence their cooperation and the kinds of services they are willing to offer (Corrigan, 2004). Perceived consistency in their views on these issues may be a catalyst for more inter-agency cooperation and the development of community-centered approaches to depression in women in rural areas.

Stressful life events, work overload and responsibilities, and inequalities in their social and economic status impact women's mental health (Judd et al., 2002; Mazure, Keita, & Blehar, 2002; Mirowsky, 1996). Among the characteristics of rural living that can contribute to depression in women are economic instability, geographic and social isolation, traditional beliefs about the roles of women, and family and social responsibilities (American Psychological Association, 2002; Carruth & Logan, 2002; Graveline, 1990). Limited occupational choices, adult education and job training opportunities, and child care resources also impact on the socioeconomic and health status of rural women (Richardson, 1988).

Epidemiological studies show that the majority of individuals with symptoms of depression are not being reached by current mental health services (Blazer, Kessler, McGonagle, & Swartz, 1994). Depressed women who reside in rural areas are less likely to obtain treatment compared to those in urban centers (Fox et al., 2001). Lack of transportation and knowledge about services, and the stigma associated with seeking mental health services contribute to access difficulties (Campbell, Gordon, & Chandler, 2002; National Institute of Mental Health, 2000; Raingruber, 2002). Even when basic health and mental health services are publicly funded, women often can't afford the ancillary costs (e.g., of transportation, child care) to make use of them (Scattolon & Stoppard, 1999).

Rural areas also have less resources and services available for the assessment and treatment of mental disorders. Mental health care professionals tend to be concentrated in urban areas (Canadian Psychological Association, 1999; Merwin, Hinton, Dembling, & Stern, 2003). Thus, community residents are often required to receive psychological services from primary care physicians who may not be adequately trained to recognize and treatmental illness (Scheffler & Zazzali, 1998; Telford, Hutchinson, Jones, Rix, & Howe, 2002). Professionals may be trained according to urban models of service delivery, which could be inappropriate for rural settings (Wagenfeld & Buffum, 1983).

It is also important to consider the appropriateness of mental health services to treat depression in women. For example, Hughes and McCormack (2000) found that women viewed the formal mental health care system (e.g., doctors, therapists) in Nova Scotia difficult to use, not affordable, and often irrelevant to their needs. Traditional treatments (e.g., medication) may not be the most effective or suitable forms of assistance for depressed women (Gammell & Stoppard, 1999; Graveline, 1990; Hauenstein, 2003). There is concern that the use of antidepressant medication is stigmatizing, expensive, and not likely to lead to long-term solutions. Furthermore, socioeconomic stresses and deprivations are not addressed when intervention follows the medical model.

Community-centered approaches utilizing local resources and services can address socioeconomic issues and reach depressed individuals in the community who have not accessed mental health services

(Alvarez & Nicemboim, 1998; Bruce, Smith, Miranda, Hoagwood, & Wells, 2002). They are cost-effective and suitable to rural communities where there is a fear of the stigma of mental illness and reluctance to go for treatment (Kenkel, 1986; Raingruber, 2002). Programs built around existing resources also help community members to become socially integrated and empowered to deal with their emotional disorders (Bergstrom, 1982; Israel, 1985; Mazure et al., 2002). More collaboration and integration among community and mental health services have been advocated as a way to improve the delivery of needed services in rural areas (Campbell et al., 2002; Hauenstein, 2003; Linzrnayer, 2003; Sears, Danda, & Evans, 1999).

Perceived consistency in the views of community service providers may promote inter-agency collaboration and the development of more accessible and appropriate services for depressed women living in rural areas. The present study examined community service providers' views of depression in rural women and their recommendations on how services might be improved. We were also interested to know whether a consistency existed between how community service providers conceptualize the problems of access and appropriateness of services for depressed rural women and their recommendations on how these services might be improved.

METHOD

Participants

Participants were obtained from a telephone directory, a community resource handbook, and through referrals from other respondents. The sample consisted of 37 participants (29 females, 8 males) from the Kings and Hants Counties of Nova Scotia. This group represented 35 community-based organizations (3 representatives surveyed were from the same group) including support groups, and community health, family, and career resource centers. To ensure that the sample of services was representative, the researchers contacted all the relevant organizations listed in the telephone directory and community resource handbook for each county. All organizations that were approached participated in the study. Many of the selected participants held positions at a senior-level, which allowed for an informed and overall view of the organization. Participants' experiences in their present profession ranged from 5 months to 41 years, with a mean of 10.85 years. The mean for service specifically in the Kings and Hants County regions was 7.23 years. The participants had a good general knowledge of depression. On average, they correctly answered (yes/no) 9 out of 10 simple questions on the topic of depression.

Measures

We developed the Community Services Survey, a semi-structured interview form, for the present study. It consists of 20 open-ended questions addressing the views of service providers on depression in women in rural communities. The first section of the survey examines the causes of depression and factors believed to contribute to the higher prevalence of depression in women. The second and third sections examine prevention and treatment services available for women in rural communities and what changes should be made to enhance services. The last section addresses the particular agency's resources and past experiences in offering services to depressed women and potential to become involved in community-based programs for them.

Procedure

Community service workers were contacted by telephone and asked if they would be willing to participate in the study. At the beginning of the interview the researchers provided an explanation of the study, described the administration procedures, and answered any questions. The participant was then asked to read and sign a consent form. The Community Services Survey was then administered. Participants' responses were also tape recorded to ensure that all information provided was captured. Upon completion of the interview, participants were debriefed verbally and were given a debriefing form to read over. They were also told that they could contact the researchers with any inquiries they might have or to obtain a copy of the results of the study. Participation took approximately one hour.

Data Analysis

Thematic analysis (Lewis, 1995), drawing on principles of grounded theory (Strauss & Corbin, 1990), was employed to analyze the responses. The responses were organized or grouped according to predominant or prevalent themes in a way that addressed both the research questions and the experiences and perceptions of the participants (Banister, Burman, Parker, Taylor, & Tindall, 1994). Data analysis began with the repeated and detailed reading of transcribed responses until the main topic areas relevant to the study were identified and survey items that addressed each of these topics were selected. For each topic area, participants' responses to items selected for that topic were read in detail to uncover predominant or recurrent themes. To develop the final themes, we identified and linked themes and responses that were common across interview accounts. All final themes were labelled and defined and prototypic excerpts were selected.

RESULTS

Thematic analysis identified themes within five main topic areas in the participants' responses. Prototypic responses are presented to illustrate each theme.

The Stresses of Depressed Women

One main theme concerned the stresses experienced by women. Stressful life circumstances, or *situational stressors*, often beyond the individual's control, were seen to contribute to risk for depression. Some of these stressors included forms of abuse (e.g., physical abuse), difficult relationships, job-related stress (e.g., unemployment) and parental stress (e.g., being a single mother). The risk for depression was believed to increase the more stressors endured at one time.

> If you have two kids, no alimony, and a woman on social assistance and your husband has done the walk or is a cheating alcoholic, what other choice do you have but to get depressed.

The *lack of financial resources* to meet basic needs were seen to affect a woman's stress level. In addition, it would likely impact her level of independence, sense of control, and self-worth, which are factors that play a role in the development of depression.

> The low-income mom might be worse because they do not get out of the house, and they are not in control of the house and there is no one else to depend on either, that tends to be a real trigger when it comes to depression.

Participants saw *societal pressures and expectations* placed on women to bear responsibilities outside the home (e.g., working full-time) as well as within (e.g., household responsibilities). If women do not live up to these ideals, their self-esteem and feelings of self-worth may be impacted.

> Social ideals-because we live in a society where women are still very much, I wouldn't go so far as to say "second-class citizens," but there is definitely still some very high social ideals on how women should behave. So, when you are outside of that mold it leads to a lot of feelings of lack of self-worth and things like that.

Stresses of Women in Rural Areas

Other stresses were particular to rural areas. Participants discussed how living in a small or rural community contributes to feelings of *isolation* and helplessness, and in turn, depression. The three sub-themes within this theme were social isolation, geographical isolation, and lack of support. *Social isolation* occurs when an individual feels isolated from other individuals, especially adult contact, which leads to a sense of loneliness. *Geographical isolation* refers to feelings of being "trapped," because an individual resides a great distance from a community or other necessities, or when there is no mode of transportation for the individual or family. *Lack of social support* may be due to lack of formal services (e.g., mental health worker, doctor) or informal resources (e.g., family, friends, members of the community) to rely on in times of need or crisis. The following excerpt captures some of these sub-themes.

> Women in rural communities are often likely to stay at home with the children while the man in the household goes out to work. Usually there is one car in the family so once that car leaves the driveway then that person is pretty much left there to fend for themselves and try to deal with everything. So, there is a lack of social contact on that side.

Many participants believed that *traditional beliefs,* such as the belief that women should stay at home and take care of the children, are more entrenched in rural areas.

> Traditional beliefs in rural communities. There is the notion that your purpose in life is to get married and have children. Many women do not have their own dreams and visions. Depending on where they live almost cements that belief.

Obstacles to the Access of Mental Health Resources

A third main theme involved obstacles to the access of mental health resources. The *inaccessibility of services* is a theme that refers to obstacles in rural areas that make it difficult to obtain care. Women may lack transportation or financial resources to access services, or may be required to travel greater distances to obtain services.

> Low income-might not be able to access counsellors or other treatments e.g., naturopathic things or eating healthier or joining the gym. They don't have the money to do those sorts of things so maybe all those things would contribute.

Participants indicated that *stigma* concerning mental health issues is another obstacle to accessing services, since it deters women from seeking help for depression.

> Lack of acceptance-you can't be as anonymous so if someone is really private they might not want other people to know that they are having difficulties. I know that rural communities can be judgmental.

Another identified concern was *lack of awareness of the signs and symptoms of depression* and when to know help is warranted. Without this understanding, women will not seek services or treatment.

> Unless someone recognizes a need, you can have all the resources out there and they don't tap into them. You can have posters and ads up and unless someone notices it and self-identifies, or has someone refer them to it, it is really difficult.

Finally, a *lack of awareness and understanding of the services* for depression also adds to the obstacles to access mental health care.

> I just think that since most people go first to their medical doctor, unless they are aware of the services, they go to their family doctor. Unless individuals have a lot of insight into their own problems or know somebody else who has been depressed, they might not necessarily go beyond what their doctors says.

Inadequate Services for Depression

Participants highlighted some of the inadequacies of mental health service delivery in rural areas. A *lack of resources* including services, supports, and professionals were seen as a major barrier to adequate care in rural areas.

> Limited resources and supports. There aren't as many as there might be in a larger area. Also, when you live in a rural area, depending on whether your families have always lived here too, you can get into different cycles-repetitive cycles in families. This may be due to lack of resources.

Participants also revealed that the current *model of treatment* may be too symptom focused, with not enough attention being paid to the causes of symptoms. Service providers often take a "quick fix" approach to treatment due to lack of funding.

> I am not a big fan of the medical model. I think that there needs to be a more holistic approach. Instead of exploring, "okay, yes you're depressed, now take this or go here and that will fix it," there needs to be more focus on the why. Instead of just fixing the symptoms, we need to look at the cause.

Recommendations for Changes in Prevention and Treatment Services

Participants made a number of recommendations for improvements in services for depressed women. They recommended that more *public education and awareness* about depression (e.g., signs and symptoms, available services) would help people to identify if someone was depressed, *when* support is needed, and *where* to go for help. Public awareness campaigns would also help to reduce stigma associated with mental illness.

> Yes, more public awareness of the services that are available so when there is early identification, that person can be assisted with inner support, to be supported to go through that.

Participants indicated that *more resources* were needed for organizations to adequately prevent and treat depression in women. If more funding were available, then organizations could hire more staff, which in turn, would reduce waitlists and enhance the quality of services.

> Need to hire a whole lot more staff. When you have a caseload of 80-100 people minimum, and maximum of up to 200, how can one person possibly deal with all those problems of all those

> families-because that is just not one person, that is caseloads of families. We can only band-aid the situation if there is not the staff in place.

Participants felt the need to *make services more accessible* to women in the community through offering transportation, outreach, and community-based programs.

> By moving into a position where resources are more accessible-would help to prevent a lot of crises that families are under. We have the vehicle now in a lot of communities-but there are some communities down the road that have nothing.

Finally, participants also recommended that services be more *proactive and preventative,* rather than reactive. They felt that the available services are too emergency-based and short-term focused. They suggested that more funding is needed for preventative programs since it is cost-effective and prevents future problems from occurring.

> Less emergency-based services-the "you are only going to be helped right now if you are in this dire situation." You need to help somebody before they get into that dire situation.

DISCUSSION

Thematic analyses identified five main topic areas in the participants' conceptualizations of depression and the services available for rural women. Many of these findings are corroborated by other research. The first main topic area described the various stressors and challenges that women faced that contribute to their depression. Previous studies have also shown that various community groups and service providers recognize the importance of psychosocial stresses in the development of depression (Jorm, Korten, Jacomb, Rodger, & Pollitt, 1997; Lauber, Falcato, Nordt, & Rossler, 2003). A second main topic related to stresses associated with rural living that increase a woman's risk for depression. These findings are consistent with other studies that found isolation and traditional beliefs about the roles of women to be characteristics of rural settings that make women more vulnerable to depression (Graveline, 1990). The third main topic focused on the obstacles faced by rural women to access mental health resources. Stigma, lack of knowledge, as well as inaccessibility of services have been recognized as delaying the seeking and receiving of treatment for mental problems, especially in rural areas (Logan et al., 2004; National Institute of Mental Health, 2000). A fourth main topic related to the lack of adequate and appropriate mental health services available in rural areas. Other studies have also found the lack of adequate services to be a major problem for depressed rural women (Hauenstein, 2003; Herzig & Murphy, 1997). In addition, traditional approaches to mental health care have been critiqued for generally overlooking the societal components of emotional distress (Gammell & Stoppard, 1999).

The fifth main topic identified the service providers' recommendations for changes in prevention and treatment and included the need for education and awareness campaigns, more resources, easier access to services, and more proactive and preventative services. These recommendations were generally consistent with their views of the societal sources of depression, access problems, and the lack of appropriate ser vices in rural communities. Similarly, Hughes and McCormack (2000) have reported on the need to educate the public on the transition signs to depression and appropriate interventions. Additionally, women in their study expressed the need for more timely services, accessible child care, and transportation. Our participants recommended that available services should be proactive, preventative, and resource-based, rather than reactive, short-term, and symptom-focused. Overall, these community service providers seemed to consider that interventions are more helpful when they are congruent with the cause of the problem, as has been found in previous research (see Iselin & Addis, 2003).

The results of this study support the need for alternative and community-centered approaches that address the socioeconomic and emotional needs of depressed women in rural areas. Formal treatment services need to be enhanced with other vital supports and community resources (Raingruber, 2002). As Hughes and McCormack (2000) have pointed out, it is important to match depressed women's needs with appropriate intervention strategies. For example, one could tap into resources available in the community (e.g., transportation and recreational programs) that could decrease women's stresses and isolation. In addition, more use of informal care and resources, which tends to be acceptable to rural women (Hauenstein, 2003), would help to bypass the stigma of mental disorders so that more women would seek help.

Some limitations of this study must be noted. First, the sample was primarily comprised of Caucasian females from a specific region of rural Nova Scotia, and thus, the findings of this study may not be generalizable to other areas. Also, the use of qualitative data in research has been critiqued for the risk of bias. This limitation, however, likely had little effect on the themes that were highlighted. All participants surveyed were experienced professionals and had a good basic knowledge of depression. Furthermore, participants were given the opportunity and freedom to express their views. Therefore, the methodology allowed for an in-depth analysis of the issues and likely yielded significant and relevant information.

In conclusion, these community workers recognized that effective treatment of depression in women in rural areas faces a number of challenges. Although there was a consistency between what they saw as the needs and stresses of depressed women and the types of intervention and preventative approaches required to remedy them, they felt that appropriate interventions were generally lacking for these women. There was also congruence in their recognition of the obstacles to access to effective interventions and services for depressed women and the types of remedies they recommended. Although overall the views of these community workers present a sobering picture with regard to the availability of effective interventions for depressed women in rural communities, the consistency in their views and attitudes does indicate a promising foundation for change. More integration of formal and informal services has been recognized as a way to meet the challenges of rural health service delivery (Linzmayer, 2003). It is important to make service providers aware of the consistencies in their views. More awareness of the consistencies in their views might act as an incentive for more inter-agency cooperation and the development of community-centered approaches to the problems of depression in women in rural communities.

REFERENCES

Alvarez, H. F., & Nicemboim, E. (1988). Prevention of mental disorders: Steps toward community interventions. *Journal of Community Psychology*, *26*, 205-217.

American Psychological Assocation, RuralPsych. (2002). The behavioral health care needs of rural women. Online: http://www.apa.org/rural/ruralwomen.pd.

Banister, P., Burman, E., Parker, I., Taylor, M., & Tindall, C. (1994). *Qualitative methods in psychology: A research guide*. Philadelphia, PA: Open University Press.

Bergstrom, D. A. (1982). Collaborating with natural helpers for delivery of rural mental health services. *Journal of Rural Community Psychology*, *3*, 5-26.

Blazer, D. G., Kessler, R. C., McGonagle, K. A., & Swartz, M. C. (1994). The prevalence distribution of major depression in a national community sample: The National Comorbidity Survey. *American Journal of Psychiatry, 151*, 979-986.
Bruce, M. L., Smith, W., Miranda, J., Hoagwood, L., & Wells, K. B. (2002). Community-based interventions. *Mental Health Services Research, 4,* 205-214.
Campbell, C. D., Gordon, M. C., & Chandler, A. A. (2002). Wide open spaces: Meeting mental health needs in underserved rural areas. *Journal of Psychology and Christianity, 21*, 325-332.
Canadian Psychological Association. (1999). *Geographical locations survey of registered psychologists in Canada.* Author: Ottawa.
Carruth, A. K., & Logan, C. A. (2002). Depressive symptoms in farm women: Effects of health status and farming lifestyle charaeteristics, behaviors and beliefs. *Journal of Community Health, 27*, 213-228.
Corrigan, P. (2004). How stigma interferes with mental health care. *American Psychologist*, 59, 614-625.
Fox, J. C., Blank, M., Rovnyak, V. G., & Barnett, R. Y. (2001). Barriers to help seeking for mental disorders in a rural impoverished population. *Community Mental Health Journal, 37*, 421-436.
Gammell, D. J., & Stoppard, J. M. (1999). Women's experiences of treatment of depression: Medicalization or empowerment? *Canadian Psychology, 40*, 112-128.
Graveline, M. J. (1990). Threats to rural women's well-being: A group response. In V. Dhruvarajan (Ed.), *Women and well-being* (pp. 169-179). Montreal: McGill-Queen's University Press.
Hauenstein, E. J. (2003). No comfort in the rural south: Women living depressed. *Archives of Psychiatric Nursing*, 77, 3-11.
Herzig, H., & Murphy, E. (1997). Rural lessons for urban services. *Journal of Mental Health (UK), 6,* 11-21.
Hughes, J., & McCormack, C. (2000). *The stories of women living with depression: Their coping strategies and resources (Report).* Halifax, NS: Maritime Centre of Excellence for Women's Health.
Iselin, M. G., & Addis, M. E. (2003). Effects of etiology on perceived helpfulness of treatments for depression. *Cognitive Therapy and Research, 27*, 205-222.
Israel, B. A. (1985). Social networks and social support: Implications for natural helper and community level interventions. *Health Education Quarterly, 12*, 65-80.
Jorm, A. F., Korten, A. E., Jacomb, P. A., Rodger, B., & Pollitt, P. (1997). Beliefs about the helpfulness of interventions for mental disorders: A comparison of general practitioners, psychiatrists and clinical psychologists. *Australian and New Zealand Journal of Psychiatry, 31*, 844-851.
Judd, F. K., Jackson, H. J., Komiti, A., Murray, G., Hodgins, G., & Fraser, C. (2002). High prevalence disorders in urban and rural communities. *Australian and New Zealand Journal of Psychiatry, 36*, 104-113.
Kenkel, M. B. (1986). Stress-coping-support in rural communities: A model for primary prevention. *American Journal of Community Psychology, 14*, 457-478.

Lauber, C., Falcato, L., Nordt, C., & Rossler, W. (2003). Lay beliefs about causes of depression. *Acta Psychiatry Scandinavia Supplement, 418*, 96-99.

Lewis, S. (1995). A search for meaning: Making sense of depression. *Journal of Mental Health, 4*, 369-382.

Linzmayer, C. (2003). Integrated human services in rural areas: A social work approach. *Rural Social Work, 8*, 25-37.

Logan, T. K., Stevenson, E., Evans, L., & Leukefeld, C. (2004). Rural and urban women's perceptions of barriers to health, mental health, and criminal justice services: Implications for victim services. *Violence and Victims, 19*, 37-62.

Mazure, C. M., Keita. B. P., & Blehar, M. C. (2002). *Summit on women and depression: Proceedings and recommendations*. Washington, DC: American Psychological Association. Online: http://www.apa.org/pi/wpo/women&depression.pdf.

Merwin, E., Hinton, I., Dembling, B., & Stern, S. (2003). Shortages of rural mental health professionals. *Archives of Psychiatric Nursing, 17*, 42-51.

Mirowsky, J. (1996). Age and the gender gap in depression. *Journal of Health and Social Behavior. 37*, 362-380.

National Institute of Mental Health. (2000). *Depression: What every woman should know*. (NIH Publication No. 00-4779). Washington, DC: National institute of Mental Health.

Raingruber, B. (2002). Client and provider perspectives regarding the stigma of and nonstigmatizing interventions for depression. *Archives of Psychiatric Nursing, 16*, 201-207.

Richardson, H. (1988). The health plight of rural women. *Women & Health, 12*, 41-54.

Scattolon, Y., & Stoppard, J. M. (1999). "Getting on with lite": Women's experiences and ways of coping with depression. *Canadian Psychology, 40*, 205-219.

Scheffler, R., & Zazzali, J. L. (1998). Supply dynamics of the mental health workforce: Implications for health policy. *Milbank Quarterly, 76*, 25-58.

Sears, S. F., Danda, C. E., & Evans, G. D. (1999) PRIME-MD and rural primary care: Detecting depression in a low-income rural population. *Professional Psychology: Research and Practice, 30*, 357-360.

Strauss, A. L., & Corbin, J. (1990). *Basics of qualitative research: Grounded theory procedures and techniques*. Newbury Park, CA: Sage.

Telford, R., Hutchinson. A., Jones. R., Rix, S., & Howe, A. (2002). Obstacles to effective treatment of depression: A general practice perspective. *Family Practice, 19*, 45-52.

Wagenfeld, M. O., & Buffum. W. E. (1983). Problems in, and prospects for, rural mental health services in the United States. *International Journal of Mental Health, 12*, 89-107.

Index

For Product Safety Concerns and Information please contact our EU
representative GPSR@taylorandfrancis.com
Taylor & Francis Verlag GmbH, Kaufingerstraße 24, 80331 München, Germany

www.ingramcontent.com/pod-product-compliance
Ingram Content Group UK Ltd.
Pitfield, Milton Keynes, MK11 3LW, UK
UKHW021247190926
475569UK00002BA/46
* 9 7 8 0 7 8 9 0 3 6 6 2 9 *